Mourad BOUKHELOUA
Mouhamed BERREHAL
Toufik IAICHE ACHOUR

CORONARY SPASM

Mourad BOUKHELOUA
Mouhamed BERREHAL
Toufik IAICHE ACHOUR

CORONARY SPASM

ScienciaScripts

Imprint

Any brand names and product names mentioned in this book are subject to trademark, brand or patent protection and are trademarks or registered trademarks of their respective holders. The use of brand names, product names, common names, trade names, product descriptions etc. even without a particular marking in this work is in no way to be construed to mean that such names may be regarded as unrestricted in respect of trademark and brand protection legislation and could thus be used by anyone.

Cover image: www.ingimage.com

This book is a translation from the original published under ISBN 978-620-6-71268-8.

Publisher:
Sciencia Scripts
is a trademark of
Dodo Books Indian Ocean Ltd. and OmniScriptum S.R.L publishing group

120 High Road, East Finchley, London, N2 9ED, United Kingdom
Str. Armeneasca 28/1, office 1, Chisinau MD-2012, Republic of Moldova, Europe
Printed at: see last page
ISBN: 978-620-7-65835-0

FOREWORD

Medicine is a constantly evolving field, where every discovery, every advance, every step forward counts. It is in this spirit of progress and quest for knowledge that this book was written.

Coronary spasm, although less well known than other cardiovascular diseases, is a subject of crucial importance. It is a condition that can have serious, even fatal, consequences, and requires thorough understanding and proper management.

This book is the result of many years of research, observation and clinical experience. It aims to provide a clear and concise understanding of coronary spasm, its causes, symptoms, diagnosis and treatment.

It is aimed at healthcare professionals who want to learn more about the subject, as well as patients and their families who want to understand this condition better.

As you read through these pages, you will discover not only the medical aspects of coronary spasm, but also the human challenges associated with it.

This book is dedicated to you, the reader. May you find in it the answers you seek, and perhaps even more.

TABLE OF CONTENTS

INTRODUCTION

Coronary heart disease is one of the most common cardiovascular diseases affecting the world's population. It is the leading cause of death in both developed and developing countries. Its basic pathophysiological mechanism is simple: a mismatch between myocardial oxygen supply and demand, leading to more or less extensive ischaemia, manifested by stable or unstable angina, myocardial infarction or sudden cardiac death.

Once considered an exclusively atherosclerotic disease, where under the influence of cardiovascular risk factors such as smoking, diabetes and dyslipidaemia, an accumulation of cholesterol in the coronary artery wall (the atherosclerotic plaque) causes a reduction in the internal lumen, resulting in imbalance and symptoms. An accumulation of cholesterol in the coronary artery wall (the atherosclerotic plaque) causes a reduction in the internal lumen, resulting in imbalance and symptoms. In addition, thromboembolic phenomena associated with rupture of this plaque exacerbate the imbalance and precipitate acute coronary syndromes (ACS).Today we know that this understanding is true, but it is incomplete because it does not explain certain clinical facts, such as infarction in fasting subjects with no risk factors and healthy coronary arteries or no evidence of plaque rupture or erosion. In the fourth universal definition of myocardial infarction(1) , the European Society of Cardiology refers to four types according to aetiology: type one is secondary to atherosclerosis, whereas type two covers all the imbalances between myocardial oxygen supply and demand responsible for acute myocardial ischaemia:

• Reduced myocardial perfusion due to fixed coronary atherosclerosis without plaque rupture,
• A spasm of the coronary artery,
• Coronary microvascular dysfunction (which includes endothelial dysfunction, smooth muscle cell dysfunction and dysregulation of sympathetic innervation),
• Coronary embolism,
• Dissection of the coronary artery with or without intramural haematoma,
•Other mechanisms reducing oxygen supply such as severe

bradyarrhythmia, respiratory failure with severe hypoxaemia, severe anaemia and hypotension/shock ;

• Or increased myocardial oxygen demand due to sustained tachyarrhythmia or severe hypertension with or without left ventricular hypertrophy.

Over the last decade, our understanding of the pathophysiology of coronary artery disease (CAD) has evolved remarkably, allowing us to recognise that other aetiologies, such as coronary spasm, are responsible for a number of clinical manifestations.

We will review this particular entity, coronary spasm, its pathogenesis and clinical implications, and we will conclude with an illustration of a highly instructive clinical case.

HISTORY OF CORONARY ARTERY SPASM

The idea that coronary spasm may be a cause of ischaemic heart disease has been around for over a century now. It was first put forward by William Osler(2) in 1910 following observations on a series of patients presenting with paroxysmal angina pectoris and sudden death:

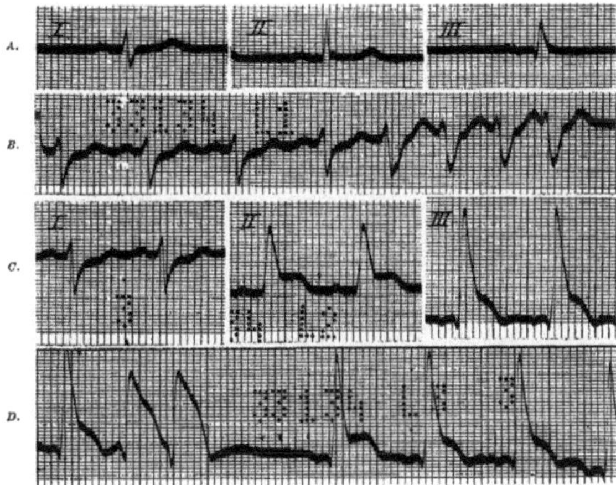

Figure 1: "Case 5. A, Standard electroenrdiogram. B, Lead I taken during the early stages of a spontaneous attack of anginal pain. C, Standard electrocardiogram taken at the height of the attack. D, Lead III, showing ventricular extrasystoles of mono-phasic outline". (3)

"The coronary arteries are not terminal arteries in the Cohnheim sense, and disease of their branches is not necessarily associated with angina. And in a few fatal cases no lesions are found; we must accept the fact that angina pectoris can kill without signs of obvious heart or blood vessel disease." Subsequently, and in the same analysis, he reported similarities between this form of angina pectoris and the phenomena observed during attacks of Raynaud's syndrome. He therefore concluded that coronary spasm was at the origin of these disorders, and here again he said: "By spasm, I mean a persistent contraction leading to ischaemia, with disruption of the function of the parts supplied"(2). A little later, in 1941 Wilson et al(3) presented a number of cases (five in number) of spontaneous or provoked angina pectoris in which per-critical electrocardiograms showed changes in the shape of the ventricular complexes "comparable in magnitude and nature to those which occur during the first few hours following the sudden occlusion of a large coronary artery"(Fig. 1). They put forward an interesting theory regarding the pathophysiology of the condition: "The pronounced electrocardiographic changes that sometimes occur during a paroxysm of angina pectoris indicate that the disruption of coronary circulation that occurs in this condition is sometimes as great as that produced by the sudden occlusion of a major coronary artery. Attacks of anginal pain may occur, accompanied by profound alterations in the electrocardiogram, in circumstances that force us to assume that the myocardial ischaemia that accompanies them is due to a change in the calibre of the coronary arteries affected, rather than to an increase in the workload of the heart alone. Nicotine or another component of cigarette smoke sometimes induces a 'spasm'.

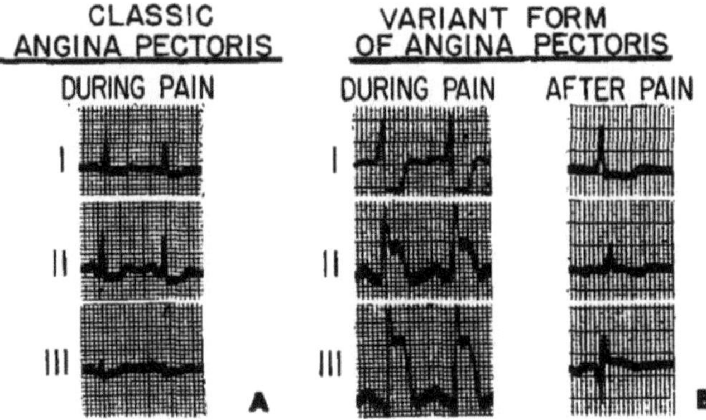

Figure 2: Comparison of the electrocardiographic characteristics of classic angina pectoris and its variant. As described by Prinzmetal (4) in patients suffering from angina pectoris"(3).

In 1959 Prinzmetal et al(4) first clearly drew attention to a group of patients with spontaneous resting angina in whom the postulated mechanism of transmural myocardial ischaemia When he described a particular form of this angina, described at the time as a "variant of angina pectoris", he found that, unlike the classic angina described by Heberden, which combines :

•Pain caused by increased cardiac workload and relieved by rest or the administration of nitroglycerine

•An electrocardiogram performed during the pain, which generally shows ST-segment depression in the standard leads without reciprocal elevation.

In this variant of angina pectoris, the pain occurs when the subject is at rest or during ordinary activity during the day or night. It is not provoked by exertion. During an attack, the ST segment is transiently and often remarkably elevated and there are reciprocal ST depressions in the standard leads (Fig. 2). Attacks almost always end spontaneously, but if they are prolonged, they can lead to death"(4).

Later on, this angina pectoris characterised by ST segment elevation, previously considered a rare entity and defined as a form of angina pectoris, became a form of angina pectoris.
This "variant" angina by Prinzmetal and colleagues has become a frequent observation since patients with recurrent attacks of angina pectoris at rest are systematically subjected to continuous electrocardiographic monitoring in coronary care units. In 1978, an article by Maseri et al(5) described the characteristics of 138 patients with "variant" angina observed in his institution over the previous 7 years (80 with angina pectoris only at rest, 58 with angina pectoris on exertion and at rest) and the results of diagnostic studies carried out on selected groups of these patients. Firstly, he was able to show that the problem lies, contrary to what has hitherto been accepted, in the reduction in perfusion without any increase in the haemodynamic determinants of myocardial demand. Thallium scintigraphy performed on 32 patients revealed a massive and localised regional reduction in myocardial perfusion during S-T segment elevation. Coronary angiography revealed no significant stenosis in 8 patients and monotruncular, bi- or tri-stenosis in 38, 34 and 26 patients, respectively. Angiography of the 37 patients studied during angina revealed a severe coronary vasospasm involving vessels of extremely variable extent of atherosclerosis. Severe arrhythmias occurred in 27 patients and myocardial infarction in 28. In all, five patients died within a month of admission to hospital.

Thus, he concludes that the "variant" form of angina represents only one aspect of a continuous spectrum of acute vasospastic myocardial ischaemia that can be observed in virtually all phases of ischaemic heart disease. And that:

•Vasospastic myocardial ischaemia can occur in the presence of an extremely variable degree of coronary atherosclerosis in patients with or without myocardial infarction and with or without typical exertional angina.

•Vasospastic myocardial ischaemia can also be characterised by depression of the S-T segment.

•Transient vasospastic myocardial ischaemia may be accompanied by chest pain or remain asymptomatic and progress to myocardial infarction and sudden death.

The authors of this article defined coronary artery spasm as "local segmental smooth muscle hyperresponsiveness secondary to a variety of stimuli that produce only mild constriction in non-spastic segments of the coronary arteries".

In 1981, using quantitative angiography and a model of adrenergic stimulation, it was demonstrated that coronary spasm was only localised in the region of pre-existing coronary atheroma. Brown et al. called this situation "hyper-reactive stenosis"(6).

Just over ten years later, a study by bugiardini et al(7) looked at the response of coronary arteries to spasm-inducing stimuli in a subgroup of patients with no or minimal coronary artery disease (< 30% stenosis) with objective signs of myocardial ischaemia. Out of twenty-five patients, ten had variant angina and fifteen syndrome X. Blood flow in the great cardiac vein, aortic pressure and changes in coronary artery diameter were measured at rest and 2 to 4 minutes after hyperventilation. The same procedure was repeated after sublingual administration of 0.3 mg nitroglycerin in eight patients (four with syndrome X and one with syndrome X). four of a "variant" of angina). At the end of this experiment, they found that hyperventilation induced a diffuse reduction in the diameter of the epicardial coronary trunks, which was marginal in control patients (9±4%) and those with coronary artery disease (5 ± 3%), but severe (p < 0.001) in those with variant angina (28 ± 14%) or syndrome X (25 ± 13%). Concomitant determination of coronary blood flow showed significant decreases (p < 0.001) in patients with variant angina (25 ± 11%) and syndrome X (28 ± 10%), but not in control patients (5 ± 8%) or those with coronary artery disease (4 ± 5 %). These results indicate that vasoconstrictor stimuli can trigger a diffuse abnormal response of epicardial and resistance vessels in some patients with chest pain and angiographically normal coronary arteries. Patients with such diffuse vasoconstrictor abnormalities are considered to have a single pathogenic entity with a spectrum of ECG manifestations ranging from depression to ST-segment elevation.

This study highlighted two important facts:

•Coronary spasticity can occur in patients without atherosclerotic lesions, who may present with symptoms of stable or unstable angina. Despite diffuse epicardial coronary vasoconstriction, the microcirculation remains the main culprit, as indicated by measurements of coronary blood flow in the coronary sinus. In some cases, functional abnormalities may be exclusive to the small or large arteries; in other cases, all components of the coronary tree may be involved.
•Endothelial dysfunction could in fact be responsible for a non-specific increase in the response to all vasoconstrictive stimuli.

More recent data indicate that endothelial dysfunction is significantly associated with a diffuse epicardial vasoconstrictor response to acetylcholine and a greater number of adverse cardiovascular events(8).

The term 'vasospastic angina' was officially coined by the Japanese Circulation Society in 2010(9). As the authors point out in their recommendations, it was perhaps time to revise the paradigm that has existed since 1959 of a single form of angina caused by a spasm of the the coronary artery and producing a transient ST-segment elevation, i.e. the variant of angina. A coronary artery may be partially occluded or diffusely narrowed by a spasm causing anginal attacks even with ST-segment depression. The guidelines state that "these pathological conditions should be collectively referred to as vasospastic angina". Variant angina, characterised by ST-segment elevation during angina attacks, is a type of vasospastic angina.

ANATOMY OF THE CIRCULATION CORONARY

The coronary arteries (CA) supply the myocardium with oxygenated blood; this is a crucial stage in the functioning of the heart and, subsequently, in the homeostasis of the body. They branch out and encircle the heart, covering its surface with a network of lace-like structures. The word coronary comes from the Latin word coronarius, meaning "belonging to a crown". In cross-section, the coronary vessels resemble an inclined, inverted crown, wrapped around the roots of the great vessels.

I. ANATOMY MACROSCOPIC

A. Origins of the coronary arteries

The coronary arteries arise from the aortic sinuses. The initial part of the aortic root, which houses the leaflets of the aortic valve, is occupied by the aortic sinuses, also known as the sinuses of Valsalva. The aortic sinuses extend beyond the upper edge of the cusp and form a well-defined, complete and circumferential sinotubular ridge when viewed from the aortic side. Depending on their position, these sinuses are known as the anterior, left posterior and right posterior aortic sinuses. The right coronary artery (RCA) arises from the anterior coronary sinus and the left common trunk (LCT) from the left posterior aortic sinus. In clinical terminology, the anterior, left posterior and right posterior sinuses are often referred to as the right, left and non-coronary sinuses respectively(10), as described by Nomina Anatomica(11). It should be noted that this description refers to the fetal arrangement of the heart prior to clockwise rotation and not to the adult, where the corresponding positions are anterior, left posterior and right posterior(12).

In around 50% of humans, a "third coronary artery" (conical artery) arises from a separate ostium in the right sinus. Other smaller ostia may be found in the right sinus, giving rise to multiple right ventricular branches. Up to five distinct coronary ostia have been described(13).If the aorta contains only two cusps or one cusp instead of the usual three, the location of the coronary ostia is generally the same as if the valve were tricuspid rather than bicuspid or unicuspid(14).The coronary arteries originate in the aortic root, the orifices generally being located at the sino-tubular junction, with a variability of up to 2.5 mm (5). The right and left coronary arteries arise perpendicular to the aorta.

With the aim of determining the origin of the coronary arteries, Michela Muriago(15) examined the coronary arterial orifices and their relationship with the aortic valve to determine the range of normality in 23 autopsied adults free of cardiac pathology. The left coronary artery arises in the left posterior aortic sinus (of Valsalva) in 16 (69%) specimens, above the sinutubular junction in five (22%) and at the junction in two (9%). The right coronary artery originated in the anterior aortic sinus in 18 (78%) specimens, above the junction in three (13%), and at the junction in two (9%). An accessory coronary orifice was found in the anterior aortic sinus in 17 (74%) specimens, while a third orifice in this sinus was found in five hearts. Coronary arterial orifices are usually located in the aortic sinuses below the sinutubular junction, but are rarely centrally located. Accessory coronary orifices are present in the majority of anterior aortic sinuses.

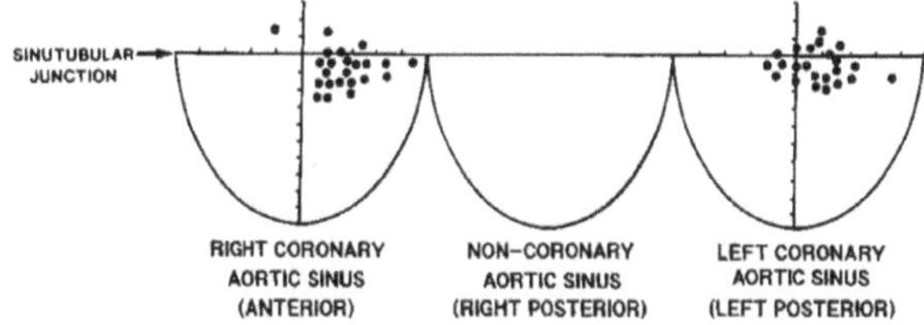

Figure 3: Diagram showing the locations of the coronary ostia (dots) in relation to the sinutubular junction and the apposition zones between the adjacent leaflets. The appearance is that of an anterior view of the aorta opened flat after a vertical incision of its anterior wall (14).

In another series published in 2010, Joshi SD(10) sought to describe the normal and variant anatomy of coronary artery ostia in Indian subjects, in order to He conducted a cadaveric study in a random population: one hundred and five heart samples were dissected, and the number of ostia and their position in the respective sinuses were studied, along with their vertical and circumferential deviations. The heights of the cusps and ostia in relation to the bottom of the sinus were measured. He found the following results: no ostia were present in the pulmonary artery or non-coronary sinus. The number of ostia in the aortic sinuses varied from 2 to

5; multiple ostia were mainly observed in the anterior sinus. The majority of ostia were located below the sinutubular crest (89%) and at or above the superior margin of the cusps (84%). Left ostial openings were predominantly centrally located (80%), while right coronary ostia were often displaced towards the right posterior aortic sinus (59%).

The results of these two series and others show that the typical configuration consists of two coronary arteries, arising respectively from the left and right aortic or coronary sinuses, in the proximal ascending aorta. The preferred location of the ostia was within the sinus and above the cusps, but below the sino-tubular crest. These are the only two branches of the ascending aorta.

B. Route and branches of division

The left coronary network

Usually, a single orifice is located in the left aortic sinus, the plane of which is inclined so that the ostium of the left coronary artery is superior and posterior to that of the right coronary artery(16).

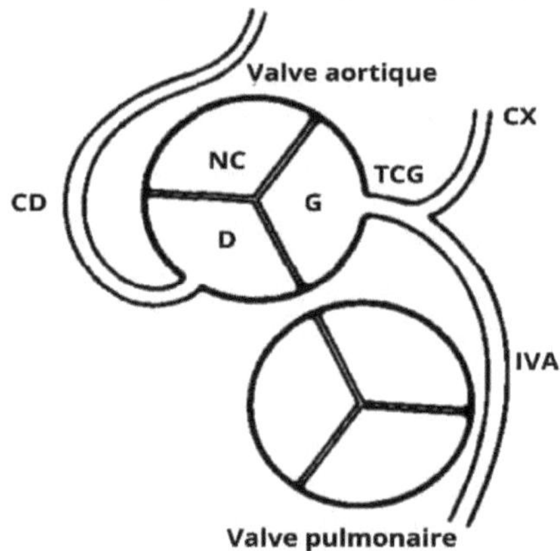

Figure 4: Origins of coronary arteries (14)

It originates in the common trunk, which passes between the pulmonary trunk and the left atrium in the subepicardial fatty tissue, and is generally between 1 and 25 mm long(13). It then continues its course in the upper part of the anterior interventricular groove, where it bifurcates into two terminal branches: the anterior interventricular and the circumflex. It does not usually branch further, but may rarely give rise to the sino-atrial nodal artery(17).

It should be noted that this common trunk may be completely absent, i.e. the anterior interventricular (AIV) and circumflex (CX) arteries arise independently of the left aortic sinus.

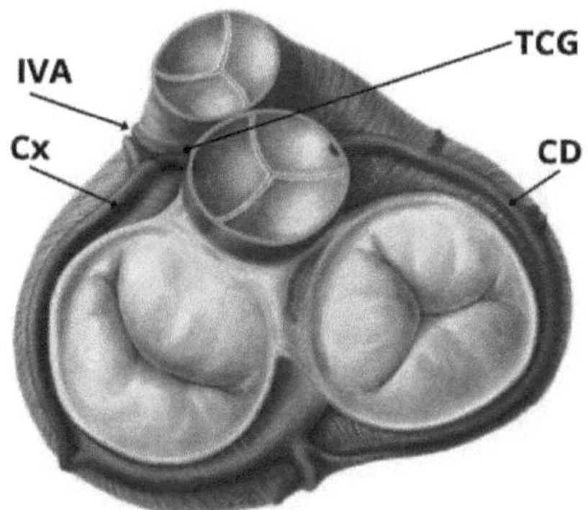

Figure 5: Relationship of the left common trunk to the pulmonary artery. TCG: left common trunk, IVA: anterior interventricular, CX: circumflex, CD: right coronary (16)

The anterior interventricular artery passes through the interventricular septum, is usually 10 to 13 cm long and gives rise to branches that penetrate the septum (septal perforators), and diagonals for irrigation of the anterolateral free wall of the left ventricle, then passes towards the apex into the anterior interventricular groove. It supplies a large part of the ventricular septum, including the right and left branches of the myocardial conduction system bundle, the anterior and apical parts of the left ventricle and the anterolateral papillary muscle of the mitral valve. The circumflex artery (the second daughter branch of the TCG) passes under the left atrium to reach the left atrioventricular groove. It varies according to dominance, but is usually around 6 to 8 cm long. It gives so-called marginal branches for irrigation of the lateral wall of the LV. In some cases, it also gives a branch behind the aorta to the superior vena cava, so that it can supply the sinus node(18). The luminal diameters of the main left coronary arteries in adults are as follows: TCG: 2.0-5.5 mm (mean 4 mm); IVA: 2.0-5.0 mm (mean 3.6 mm); circumflex: 1.5-5.5 mm (mean 3.0 mm)(13). An intermediate artery known as a bisector may arise between the two, so that the left common trunk becomes trifurcated (in around 15% of cases).

The right coronary

The dominant right coronary artery is usually about 12-14 cm long, runs horizontally along the right atrioventricular groove and gives

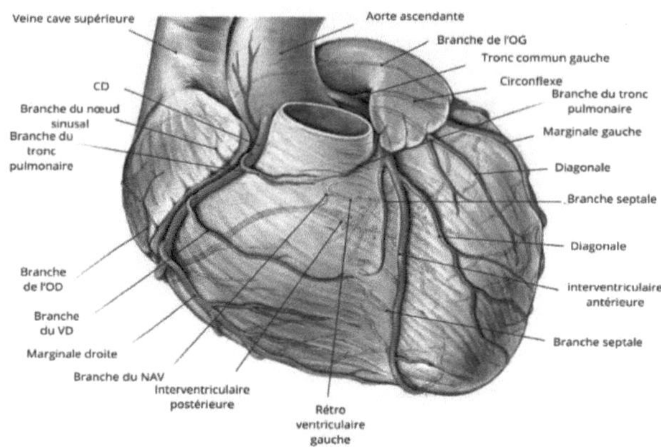

Figure 6. Complete coronary arterial system (18)

It originates at the right marginal border, supplying the right ventricle. It then continues in the same sulcus to the lower surface of the heart, where it turns forwards at the level of the crest to give the posterior interventricular artery (PVI) in around 90% of the human population (the latter arises from the CX in the remaining 10%), heading towards the apex on the posterior or diaphragmatic surface of the heart(19). It supplies the posterior myocardium of both ventricles, the posterior third of the interventricular septum and the posteromedial papillary muscle of the mitral valve. Its diameter varies between 1.5-5.5 mm, with an average of 3.2 mm(13). Although the VIA and circumflex generally decrease in diameter as they extend from the left main bifurcation, the right coronary artery remains relatively constant in diameter until just before the origin of its posterior interventricular branch.

The sub-epicardial coronary arteries run along the surface of the heart, embedded in varying amounts of sub-epicardial fat. Portions of these epicardial arteries may plunge into the myocardium and be covered over a variable length (1 to several mm) by the ventricular muscle, known as the myocardial bridge.

C. Dominance coronary

Cardiac dominance is dictated by which branch of the coronary artery gives rise to the PVI and supplies the inferior wall, and is characterised as left, right or codominance (balanced). The vessel most often originates from the right coronary artery (right dominance), the left circumflex artery (left dominance) or both (codominance).It is estimated that 70-80% of the population has a dominant right heart, with the PVI coming from the right coronary artery. Approximately 5-10% of the population has a dominant left heart, with the PVI coming from the circumflex artery, and approximately 10-20% is co-dominant, with the PVI supplied by both the left circumflex artery and the right coronary artery(20).

D. Coronary veins

The venous system of the cardiac muscles runs parallel to the coronary arteries. Venous drainage of the left ventricular myocardium is completed by the interventricular vein and the great cardiac vein, which drains into the coronary sinus, located in the posterior right atrioventricular groove, which in turn empties into the right atrium. The anterior cardiac veins are responsible for draining blood from the right ventricular myocardium directly into the right atrium

.

II. HISTOLOGY OF THE CORONARY ARTERIES

Like all arteries, coronary arteries can be divided into three concentric layers:

•An inner (luminal) layer: the intima ;
•An intermediate layer: the media ;
•An outer layer: the adventitia(21).

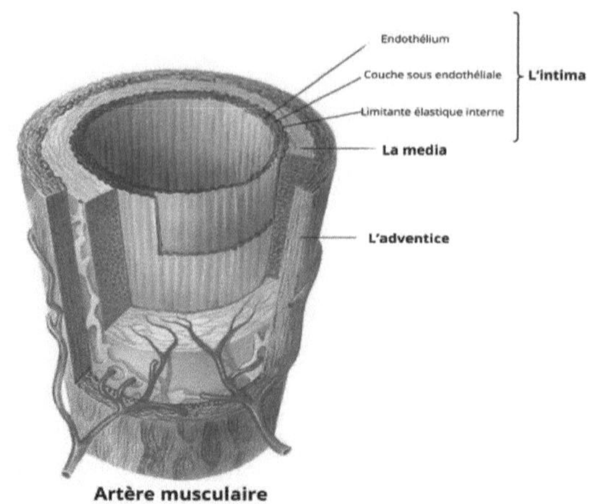

Figure 7. Histological structure of an artery (21)

A. The intima

It is made up of a layer of endothelial cells, a subendothelial layer containing connective tissue and smooth muscle cells. helium is a specialised epithelium which forms a smooth luminal wall and a selective diffusion barrier between the blood and the other layers of the blood vessel.

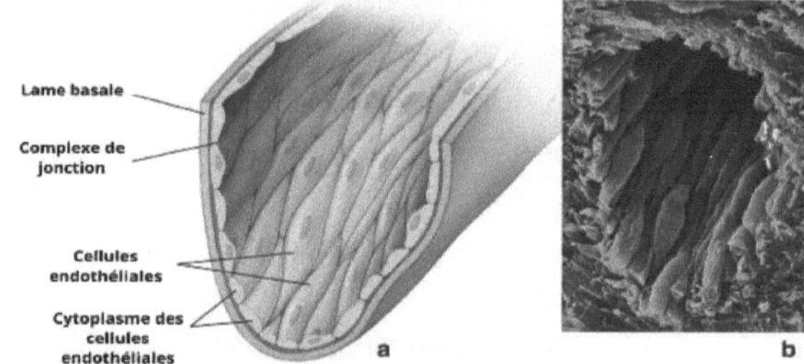

Figure 8. Schematic and scanning electron micrograph of the endothelium.

a. This diagram shows the luminal surface of the endothelium. The cells are elongated with their long axis parallel to the direction of blood flow.

b. Scanning electron micrograph showing the cells of the endothelial lining.{22} wall. Vascular endothelial cells are squamous, polygonal and elongated with the long axis in the direction of blood flow. The nuclei of endothelial cells are also elongated in the direction of blood flow(22).until recently, the endothelium was considered to be a simple barrier modulating diffusion. Current information indicates that it is, together with its basal lamina, highly differentiated to mediate and actively control the bidirectional exchange of molecules by simple and active diffusion, receptor-mediated endocytosis, transcytosis and other mechanisms(23). Endothelial cells also have a number of metabolic and endocrine functions that play a critical role in various physiological and pathological states.The intimal layer is separated from the media by a sparse subendothelial layer of connective tissue and a prominent internal elastic membrane.

B. The media

It is made up of several layers of smooth muscle cells and connective tissue (elastic fibres, collagen, proteoglycans). The quantity of The number of smooth muscle cells is greater in epicardial coronary arteries than in other elastic vessels. The media consists of 40 layers of circumferentially or helically oriented smooth muscle. The thickness of the normal media varies from 125 to 350 μm (200 μm on average). The medial layer is separated from the adventitial layer by the outer elastic membrane. The outer elastic membrane is composed of interrupted layers of elastin and is considerably thinner than the inner elastic membrane. Unmyelinated nerve axons adhere tightly to the outer edge of the outer elastic membrane(13).

C. Weeds

The adventitial layer is made up of fibrous tissue (collagen, elastic fibres) surrounded by vasa vasorum, nerves and lymphatic vessels. The collagen bundles that surround it are mainly oriented longitudinally. The orientation of the collagen and the relatively The "loose" nature of the adventitia allows continuous changes in coronary diameter. The thickness of the adventitia varies from 300 to 500 μm(13).

PHYSIOLOGY OF CORONARY CIRCULATION

Compared with the rest of the organs, the heart is considered to be very active metabolically, with the highest oxygen consumption. Indeed, we know that the average oxygen extraction by the myocardium is 60 to 70% under physiological resting conditions, which translates into a coronary venous pO2 of around 20 mm Hg. This oxygen demand is met by the coronary circulation, which is responsible for supplying blood to the myocardium and accounts for around 5% of cardiac output(24).

The coronary arteries are made up of two parts:

• A superficial epicardial part represented by the coronary trunks, which are of large calibre and responsible for conduction of blood flow.

• An intramuscular part made up of smaller vessels developing inside the myocardium; their various branches and arterioles offer higher resistance but finer control of blood flow. Adequate blood flow in the coronary vessels is essential to avoid ischaemia and maintain the integrity of myocardial tissue. Depending on the ventricular rate, contractility and pressures, the myocardial oxygen demand can be multiplied by several, and because of the high basic oxygen consumption of the myocardium, the increase in oxygen extraction is very limited because it is already at its maximum, so most of this demand has to be met by an increase in coronary flow.

Blood flow to most tissues occurs during systole due to the increase in pressure in the aorta and its distal branches. Blood flow in the coronary vessels, however, does not meet this standard and peaks during ventricular diastole. This unusual aspect results from the external compression of the coronary vessels by the myocardial tissue during systole. This compressive force is exerted more strongly in the subendocardial layers than in the epicardial region and is so strong that it leads to a total cessation or even reversal of coronary flow, particularly in the intramuscular vessels of the left ventricle more thick. When the ventricles relax during diastole, the coronary vessels are no longer compressed and normal blood flow resumes. A particular feature of the right ventricle is that it generates lower pressures to perfuse the pulmonary circulation. As a result, right ventricular pressures are much lower than the pressures exerted by the left ventricle. Perfusion of the right ventricle occurs mainly in systole, as systolic aortic pressure exceeds systolic right ventricular pressure. The right ventricle is also perfused to a lesser extent in diastole, when aortic end-diastolic pressure exceeds right ventricular end-diastolic pressure by a smaller differential(25).

I. THE DETERMINANTS OF FLOW CORONARY BLOOD FLOW

Coronary perfusion pressure (CPP) is determined by the gradient between aortic diastolic blood pressure and left ventricular end-diastolic pressure(26-28), and this gradient is vital because it is responsible for myocardial perfusion. Increasing coronary flow, either by increasing coronary perfusion pressure or by inducing coronary vasodilatation, is the principal means of increasing oxygen supply to the myocardium.

The main determinants of coronary blood flow are :

A. Aortic pressure

As with any vascular bed, the available pressure gradient is a determinant of blood flow. The heart's ability to generate systemic arterial pressure depends, of course, on adequate coronary blood flow. Aortic pressure represents the afterload of the left ventricle, and a change in aortic pressure also leads to a change in myocardial metabolism.

B. Extravascular compression of the myocardium

The ventricular myocardium generates sufficient pressure with each beat to virtually stop coronary inflow during systole. This means that most of this coronary flow occurs during diastole. If the intra myocardial (tissue) pressure during diastole is high intraventricular (cavity) pressure, particularly in the subendocardial layers of the heart, there may be compression of the coronary circulation.

C. Myocardial metabolism

As in other vascular beds, coronary circulation is controlled by local factors. An increase in cardiac metabolism is accompanied by functional coronary vasodilatation. Cardiac metabolism increases with heart rate and the development of ventricular pressure.

D. Control neuronal

Coronary vessels are innervated by the parasympathetic and sympathetic divisions of the autonomic nervous system. Parasympathetic activation causes coronary vasodilation, while the direct effect of sympathetic activation is vasoconstriction.

II. SELF-REGULATION OF CORONARY FLOW

It is important to note that CPAP is not the only determinant of coronary blood flow. Coronary autoregulation, as defined by Johnson: "the intrinsic tendency of an organ to maintain a constant blood flow despite variations in arterial perfusion pressure"(29), therefore describes the process that allows coronary blood flow to match myocardial demand within a CPAP range of 60 to 180 mmHg(30). Coronary vasoconstriction and vasodilation are responsible for autoregulation; when CPAP is reduced, vasodilation improves flow, and the opposite is true when CPAP becomes higher(26,27).

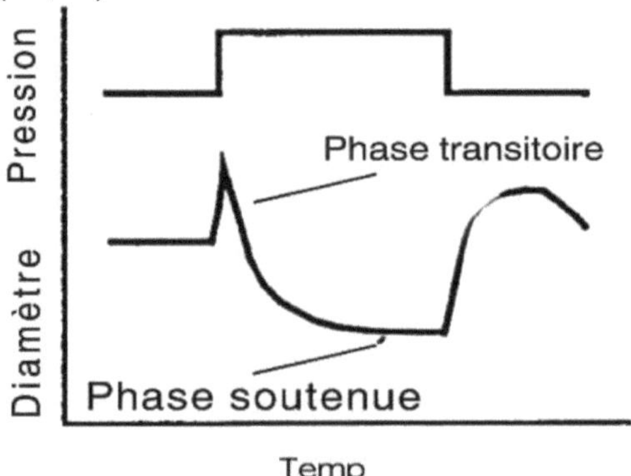

Figure 9. Myogenic behaviour: prototypical myogenic response of a cannulated arteriole to a progressive increase in pressure. (33)

This modulation of flow is not possible without a basal muscle tone, known as the vascular myogenic response, originally described by Bayliss in 1902(31), and whose work on cats, dogs and rabbits has led to the following conclusions:

•"The muscular layer of the arteries reacts, like smooth muscle in other situations, to a stretching force by contracting".

•"It also reacts to a reduction in tension by relaxing, which of course only happens when it is in a toned state".
•"These reactions are independent of the central nervous system and are myogenic in nature.
•"They are obtained both on vessels in their normal state in the body and on arteries taken a few hours after death"(31).

This myogenic response is defined as the capacity of vascular smooth muscle to contract in response to an increase in transmural force (i.e. perfusion pressure). By extension, a decrease in intravascular pressure is followed by a transient collapse in diameter followed by dilation(32). This behaviour is thought to represent the vessel's efforts to minimise wall stress, according to Laplace's law:

E. Parietal stress Pressure x rayonwall thickness

In addition, it allows a certain degree of active force to be maintained at normal intravascular pressures, i.e. the basal or myogenic 'tone', which allows microvascular resistance to be modulated in both directions by the actions of vasodilators and vasoconstrictors. Figure 9 illustrates an example of myogenic behaviour, showing the prototypical myogenic response of a cannulated arteriole to a progressive increase in pressure. After the pressure plateau, initial passive distension is followed by two phases of constriction; when the pressure plateau is released, the arteriole collapses transiently and then dilates(33).

On the basis of this relationship between vessel diameter and the extent of the myogenic response, it is thought that the myogenic response plays an important role in maintaining basal vascular tone. It is therefore in the presence of this 'background' vasomotor tone that non-myogenic factors have a bidirectional influence on the regulation of coronary flow, which is necessary to balance the supply of oxygen to the myocardium and myocardial oxidative metabolism.

Therefore, CPAP represents the pressure gradient across the coronary vasculature, while resistance is mediated by autoregulation to provide the required flow rates(34). Multiple factors are responsible for coronary vasomotricity, which occurs in autoregulation :

- Neurohormonal factors,
- Endocrine factors,
- Metabolic factors,
- Endothelium-derived factors.

A. Neurohormonal factors

The coronary vessels are among the most innervated vessels in the body, as described in the work of H. H. Woollard in 1926, when he spoke of this sympathetic and parasympathetic innervation(35).

Subsequent electron microscopy studies have shown that nerve fibres are located in the coronary vascular wall and that small arteries and arterioles contain more nerve endings than large coronary arteries(36,37). The main sympathetic trunks appear to be located in the epicardium alongside the coronary arteries, with transmural penetration to innervate the rest of the myocardium. On the other hand, the main ventricular parasympathetic pathways remain epicardial until they cross the AV groove, where vagal fibres penetrate the myocardium to localise mainly in the ventricular subendocardium(38,39).

In general, sympathetic nerves release norepinephrine, neuropeptide Y and ATP, while parasympathetic nerves release acetylcholine and vasoactive intestinal polypeptide(34).

The expression of adrenergic receptors varies throughout the coronary tree, with □1 adrenoreceptors predominantly expressed in the larger epicardial arteries, and □2 adrenoreceptors predominantly located in the microcirculation <100 µm in diameter. Activation of these receptors causes marked vasodilation (40).

The primary site for a-adrenoceptors appears to be further upstream in the coronary circulation, with many studies supporting a non-uniform distribution of a1-adrenoceptors in large arteries and a2-adrenoceptors in small arteries and large arterioles. Interestingly, functional assessment of a- and □-adrenoceptor responses to noradrenaline in isolated, pressurised coronary vessels revealed dose-dependent constriction of the vessels greater than 100 µm in diameter and dilation of vessels less than 100 µm in diameter(34). This action, described as paradoxical, seems to minimise coronary "flight" by inducing vasoconstriction of the proximal vessels with dilation of the distal vessels, but in the latest studies we have no solid evidence in favour of better blood flow to the inner layers of the myocardium or better function/metabolism with a-adrenergic coronary vasoconstriction, because this phenomenon is not as robust as many other mechanisms of coronary blood flow regulation and can be easily overridden(41).

Coronary blood flow responses to muscarinic receptor activation, via acetylcholine (Ach) administration or vagal stimulation, are highly species and concentration dependent, with experiments in most animal models and healthy human vessels demonstrating significant endothelium-dependent vasodilation in vessels ranging from 50 to 400 µm in diameter (42,43). Muscarinic coronary vasodilation has been attributed to both M1 and M2 receptors, with stimulation of M2 receptors resulting in redistribution of blood flow to the subendocardium (44,45).

B. Endocrine factors

Angiotensin II

Angiotensin II, a highly potent vasoconstrictor, is an octapeptide produced by the cleavage of angiotensin I by the converting enzyme, which is expressed in the heart and coronary endothelium. If administered intravenously, it causes a modest concentration-dependent increase in coronary blood flow mediated by peripheral vasoconstriction and an increase in systemic blood pressure with secondary stimulation of local metabolic vasodilatory mechanisms. In contrast, intracoronary administration of angiotensin II induces pronounced coronary vasoconstriction which is completely abolished by inhibition of AT1 receptors with telmisartan(34,46).

Vasopressin

The function of antidiuretic hormone (ADH) is to retain water in the body and it is also capable of causing vasoconstriction, hence its name: vasopressin. It should be noted that the pressor activity of vasopressin depends on the endothelium and seems to be linked to the diameter of the coronary artery in question, in the sense that in arteries with a diameter greater than 100 µm it causes endothelium-dependent vasodilation. In contrast, it has been shown to cause vasoconstriction in arteries less than 90 µm in diameter, as shown in the work of Meyrs et al(47) who examined the role of the endothelium in modulating responses to acetylcholine, vasopressin and thrombin and compared these responses with those observed in large epicardial vessels. They found that in the large vessels, vasopressin provokes vasodilation which is reduced by elimination of the endothelium. The same result was reported by Katusic et al (48). On the other hand, in small coronary vessels, vasopressin only produced vasoconstriction which was reinforced by the addition of haemoglobin(34,47).

Histamine

Histamine is an essential mediator in allergic and inflammatory responses. When released by immune cells, it modulates vascular tone via two distinct receptors (H1 and H2), resulting in arteriolar vasodilatation via H2 receptors, the presence of which has been demonstrated in the coronary circulation.Nakayama et al(49) in their study of the histamine response of porcine coronaries found that epicardial arteries responded to histamine with greater reductions in diameter. In contrast, they showed that resistance vessels hardly contracted at all to histamine, even at the highest concentration used to contract epicardial conductance vessels. The same observation was made by Ginsburg et al (50) who reported greater sensitivity to histamine-induced vasoconstriction in the proximal than in the distal parts of the large human coronary arteries. In humans, the H1 receptors in the coronary endothelium stimulate the release o f nitric oxide to a level sufficient to induce a coronary vasodilatation in response to exogenous histamine. However, the role of endogenous histamine in regulating coronary vascular tone in response to a physiological stimulus has not yet been demonstrated(34).

C. Factors metabolism

Vasomotor tone is determined almost exclusively by local metabolic oxygen demand. Given that the left ventricle extracts around 70-80% of the oxygen supplied by arterial blood under baseline conditions, it is essential that there are mechanisms to ensure that the left ventricle's vasomotor tone is maintained.

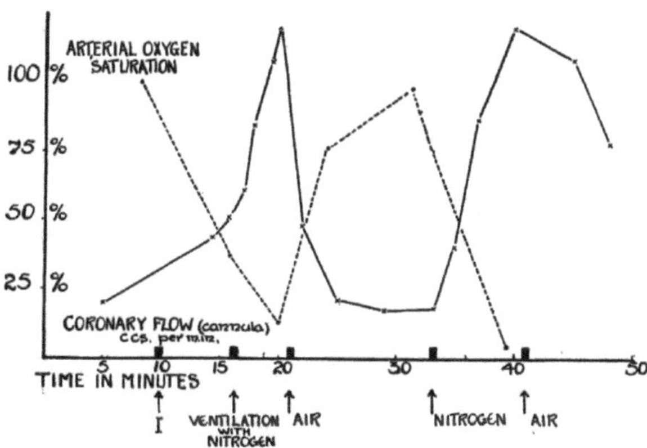

Figure 10: Effect on coronary flow of a reduction in 02 saturation in arterial blood (51)

Changes in myocardial metabolism (demand) are balanced by concordant and proportional changes in oxygen supply. These mechanisms are complex and not yet fully understood, involving several pathways and metabolites.

Role of oxygen

The role of hypoxia in increasing coronary flow has been known since the work of Hilton and Eicholtz(51) , who studied the behaviour of coronary flow in dogs as a function of oxygen saturation. following pulmonary ventilation with nitrogen causes a five-fold increase in flow compared with the baseline situation and that resuming ventilation with ambient air causes this flow to fall again (fig.10).

A role for the activation of oxygen sensors in terminal arterioles and capillaries, which initiate vasodilatory responses, has been suggested in the genesis of hypoxic vasodilation conducted from their origin to distant resistance arterioles (52-54). A role for the endothelium as a potentiator, as well as for other metabolites, has also been debated by several authors(34).

Role of potassium

Potassium has been proposed as a potential regulator of coronary blood flow, and its role in vasodilation has been known since the work of

Konold et al. In 1968(55) they demonstrated that rinsing the outside of a coronary artery with a solution containing potassium provoked vasodilatation which disappeared, giving way to vasoconstriction if the concentration was excessive (generally >20 mmol/L), since which time several studies have not produced unanimous results, leading to the conclusion that although potassium may play a transient role in the initiation of metabolic vasodilatation, it is unlikely to contribute to the increase in coronary blood flow in response to the increase in myocardial metabolism(34).

Adenosine

Berne in 1963(56) was the first to suggest a role for adenosine in the local metabolic control of coronary blood flow by conducting experiments on isolated cat hearts perfused with Tyrode's solution and on intact open-chest dog hearts. Cardiac hypoxia led to a decrease in coronary vascular resistance and the release of significant quantities of inosine and hypoxanthine (breakdown products of adenosine) by the myocardium. which proposes the powerful vasodilatory factor adenosine (a degradation product of ATP) as the main factor released by the myocardium in proportion to increases in myocardial oxidative metabolism and/or reductions in myocardial oxygenation. Increased concentrations of adenosine in the cardiac interstitium then increases coronary blood flow by activating specific receptors on coronary vascular smooth muscle cells(34).This fascinating hypothesis has not been supported by subsequent studies, which have failed to show any significant effect on coronary flow; we cite here the work of Bache et al. in 1988(57) who, in order to verify this hypothesis, examined the active hyperaemia associated with gradual treadmill exercise and coronary reactive hyperaemia in awake, chronically instrumented dogs, after intracoronary infusion of adenosine deaminase (5 units/kg/min for 10 minutes) and after blockade of adenosine receptors by 8-phenyltheophylline. They concluded that: ...although adenosine deaminase and 8-phenyltheophylline antagonised coronary vasodilation in response to exogenous adenosine and attenuated coronary reactive hyperaemia, neither agent altered coronary vasodilation associated with exercise-induced increases in myocardial oxygen demand. These results do not confirm that adenosine plays an important role in coronary vasodilation during exercise... In the same vein, Yada et al (58) in 1999 designed an experiment in which myocardial oxygen consumption was increased by cardiac stimulation. The tachycardia of the stimulation avoided the direct vascular effects of vasoconstriction mediated by a-adrenergic receptors and vasodilatation mediated by □-adrenergic receptors. They found that interstitial adenosine concentration did not reach vasoactive levels before or during adenosine receptor blockade, indicating that adenosine is not important in the local metabolic control of coronary blood flow.Taken together, these data indicate that while adenosine is capable of inducing potent vasodilation, these effects are not physiologically evident unless the oxygen supply to the myocardium is compromised (i.e. the myocardium is ischaemic)(34).

Reactive oxygen species (H2O2)

One of the most recent theories is that of reactive oxygen species. Superoxide is produced by several enzymatic systems

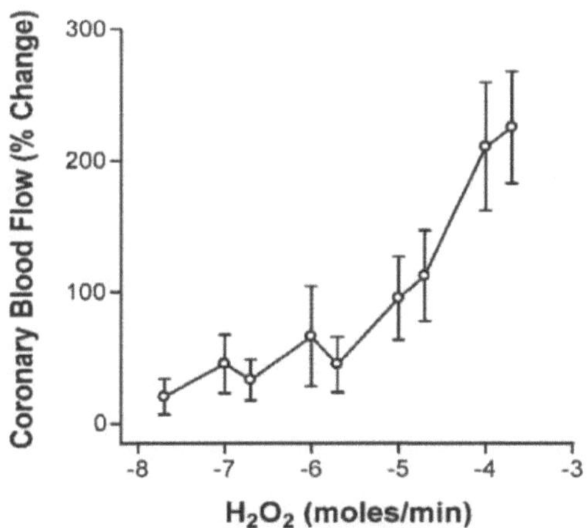

Figure 11. Intracoronary infusion of H2O2 increases blood flow in a dose-dependent manner (61).

in the cell secondary to mitochondrial respiration(59) and is converted to hydrogen peroxide (H2O2) by superoxide dismutase. H2O2 can be degraded by catalase to form H2O and an oxygen molecule(60). When administered exogenously, the vasodilatory properties of H2O2 are well known since the work of Rogers et al(61) who demonstrated in 2006 that intracoronary infusion of H2O2 increased blood flow in a dose-dependent manner (Fig. 11) with no change in heart rate or blood pressure, suggesting that the cardiovascular effects were limited to the coronary circulation. Furthermore, neither denudation of the endothelium nor inhibition of cyclooxygenase altered H2O2-induced relaxation of the arterial rings, suggesting a direct action on vascular smooth muscle and that this redox-sensitive coronary vasodilation induced by H2O2 is mediated by K channels sensitive to 4-aminopyridine. In addition, it should not be forgotten that H2O2 has a role as an endothelium-derived hyperpolarising factor which will be discussed later.

D.Factors derived from the endothelium.

Nitric oxide (NO)

Since the early 1980s, the involvement of the vascular endothelium in the regulation of arterial tone in response to several stimuli (e.g. acetylcholine, bradykinin, histamine, serotonin, etc.) has been suspected(62), this involvement being via an "endothelium-derived relaxing factor" (EDRF) which was subsequently identified as nitric oxide(63).

NO, a molecular gas, is formed enzymatically from L-arginine by three isoforms of nitric oxide synthase (NOS)(64) :

•Neuronal-type NOS (nNOS, NOS1),
•Cytokine- or macrophage-induced NOS (iNOS, NOS2),
•Endothelial-type NOS (eNOS, NOS3).

These three enzymes catalyse the conversion of L-arginine to L-citrulline, with the production of nitric oxide. Endothelial cells constitutively express eNOS, generating relatively low levels of NO which are tightly controlled by regulatory factors. In contrast, iNOS is not normally expressed, but when induced by inflammatory cytokines, it can generate large quantities of NO, far in excess of those produced by eNOS. NO is a paracrine mediator; when it is produced and released by cells, it easily penetrates the biological membranes of neighbouring cells, modulating a number of signalling cascades. Because it has an extremely short half-life, its effects are local and transient. The cellular target of NO is soluble guanylate cyclase, which when stimulated causes the synthesis of cyclic guanosine monophosphate (cGMP) from guanosine triphosphate, thereby increasing cytosolic levels of cGMP and inducing hyperpolarisation of vascular smooth muscle via the opening of K+ channels, resulting in vasodilation(65,66).

Cyclooxygenase-derived dilatation factors

These are metabolites of arachidonic acid, which is found in the plasma membrane of almost every cell in the body. Once released, it is metabolised into different substrates via the cyclooxygenase, responsible for the production of prostaglandins, which include a variety of vasoactive compounds, such as the vasodilator prostaglandin I2 (PGI2 or prostacyclin), as well as the vasoconstrictor compounds prostaglandin H2 and thromboxane A2. The vascular vasodilatory actions of prostacyclin are mediated by adenylyl cyclase/AMP activity on K+ channels. (67-69)

Endothelium-derived hyperpolarising factors

Numerous endothelium-derived hyperpolarising factors have been identified (70-74):

•The cytochrome P-450 metabolites of arachidonic acid,
•H2O2,
•Potassium,
•H2S,
•Anandamide
•Nitroxyl.

Among these factors, H2O2 is one of the most important regulators of coronary vascular tone in response to a variety of stimuli, including cyclic stretch, shear stress, and physiological agonists such as bradykinin and acetylcholine. It mediates vasodilation through direct effects on vascular smooth muscle and may facilitate amplification and/or prolongation of endothelial cell hyperpolarisation through the opening of KCa channels (71).

Endothelium-derived vasoconstrictor factors

• Endothelin-1 is the most powerful and longest-lasting vasoconstrictor. It is a peptide of 21 amino acids produced by the endothelin-converting enzyme. Binding of endothelin-1 to ETA or ETB receptors in smooth muscle leads to powerful vasoconstriction which can last for several minutes (75,76).

• Cyclooxygenase-derived constriction factors: prostaglandin H2 and thromboxane A2 produce marked vasoconstriction in the coronary circulation, but there is no significant evidence for their role in regulating coronary vascular tone under normal physiological conditions. On the other hand, numerous studies have highlighted the pathophysiological role of thromboxane A2 and serotonin in pathological conditions such as activation of the coronary arteries. platelet (77) and endothelial lesions. These factors are involved in coronary vasospasm(78).

Coronary spasm remains the main cause of myocardial ischaemia without coronary artery obstruction (INOCA)(79) , and its prevalence is difficult to estimate, varying between 3% and 95% of patients presenting with a myocardial infarction without coronary artery obstruction (MINOCA)(80) ; This large difference depends on many factors, including the clinical presentation and selection of patients in the studies, the definition and diagnostic criteria for spasm, the presence or absence of associated atherosclerotic coronary disease with all the risks of spasm being unrecognised, especially if provocation tests are not routinely performed, the ethnic origin of the patients. etc.In a study published in 2006 by Raffaele Bugiardini et al(81) to investigate outcomes and methods of risk stratification in patients with MINOCA in non-ST elevation acute coronary syndrome, angiographic data from 7656

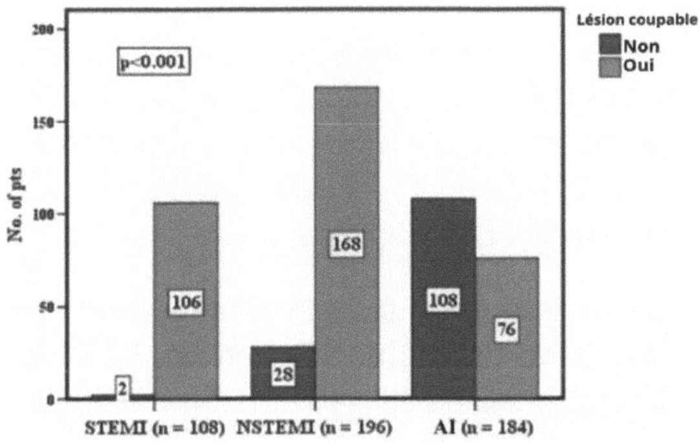

Figure 12: Distribution of the different presentations of ACS according to the presence or absence of a culprit lesion. NSTEMI non-ST-segment elevation myocardial infarction; STEMI ST-segment elevation myocardial infarction; UA unstable angina(83).

patients were pooled from 3 trials of thrombolysis in myocardial infarction (TIMI): (TIMI 11B, TIMI 16 and TIMI 22). A total of 6,955 patients had coronary obstruction and 701 had non-obstructive coronary artery disease, representing an incidence of 9.1%.In a more recent study(82) of 2,442 patients presenting with non-ST-segment elevation acute coronary syndromes with elevated troponin levels, 197 (8.8%) had MINOCA.

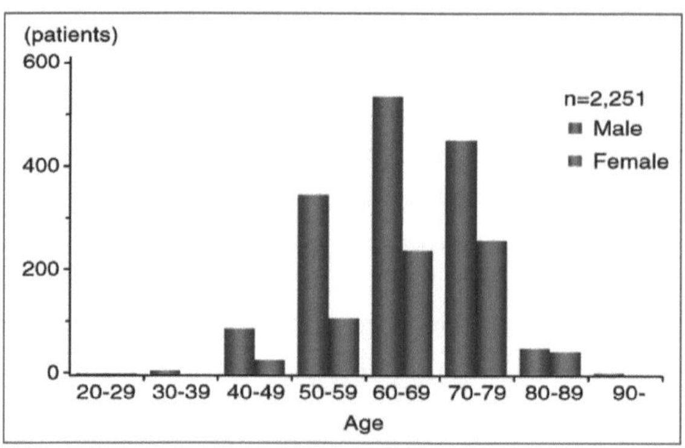

Figure 13: Age distribution of angina pectoris in the Japanese population. (84)

In another study published in 2008 by Ong et al(83), the aim of which was to assess the incidence of coronary spasm, all patients with suspected ACS who underwent coronary angiography and those without a culprit lesion had an intracoronary acetylcholine challenge test. Of 488 consecutive patients, 138 had no culprit lesion (28%). Twenty-two were ruled out for other diagnoses. ACH testing was performed in 86 of the remaining 116 patients. Coronary spasm was detected in 42 patients, representing an incidence of 49%. (Fig. 22)

Spasm is more common in men than in women, as demonstrated in a study published in Japan in 2000(84) involving 2,251 angina patients (mean age 65.2) hospitalised in 15 major cardiovascular medical institutions in Japan in 1998. We also note that the prevalence of angina in men increases with age, and that in women, the prevalence of angina in men increases with age. In women, the incidence of angina begins to rise at the average age of menopause, around 50, and gender differences in incidence no longer exist beyond the age of 80 (Fig.23). These results are similar to those found by Hung et al. in 2010(85): in a study of 722 patients who underwent diagnostic coronary angiography, 408 patients presented with coronary spasm, with a mean age of 59 ± 12 years and 69% were men. An important factor to bear in mind when attempting to explain this difference between the sexes is the particularity of the clinical manifestation in women, who are less likely to present with typical angina or to undergo angiography, and as a result underdiagnosis may be more frequent. In addition to this difference, spasm of the epicardial arteries seems to be more frequent in men and microvascular spasm in women(86).Japanese patients are much more likely to develop coronary artery vasospasm than Caucasian patients, with the risk estimated in some studies to be 3 times higher. However, no study has been able to determine whether this phenomenon is linked to genetic or environmental factors(87,88).

Finally, it is worth noting the fairly frequent association between spasm and the myocardial bridge(89), which may be explained by the fact that the increase in mechanical stress and shear forces secondary to compression in the bridge are thought to lead to endothelial dysfunction and increased susceptibility to spasm(87,90).

III. MYOCARDIAL ISCHEMIC SYNDROME

The clinical manifestation of myocardial ischaemia due to coronary spasm is chest discomfort, which is practically similar to that of stable exertional angina, in fact it reproduces its main characteristics, particularly in terms of location, irradiation and type, and is described as(91) :

• Pain localised in the chest, near the sternum, or retrosternal; but may be felt in the epigastric region; one of its main characteristics is that it is vague and cannot be indicated by a single finger(9),
• It radiates to the lower jaw or teeth, between the shoulder blades, or down either arm to the wrist and fingers.
• It feels like pressure, oppression or heaviness, sometimes like strangulation, constriction or burning.
• It may be accompanied by shortness of breath, cold sweats and discomfort, nausea, vomiting or agitation. It is a distressing pain, sometimes with a sensation of imminent death. Sometimes it is accompanied by syncope.

In fact, the clinical presentation of typical coronary spasm as described above is subject to considerable variability, which is related to the duration of the spastic episode.

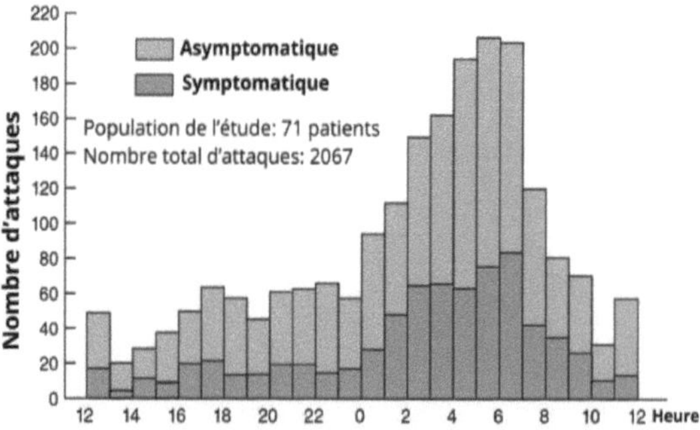

Figure 14: Diurnal variation in coronary spasm attacks (9).

Longer episodes are responsible for ACS (unstable angina, NSTEMI and STEMI) and sudden death(79). Silent ischaemia, often observed during a short episode, has been reported to be twice as frequent as angina pectoris and chest pain, which are considered to be the most common symptoms (Fig. 24)(92).

Angina attacks due to coronary spasm often persist longer than stress angina attacks due to organic lesions. They can be provoked by hyperpnoea and alcohol consumption and calmed by fast-acting nitrates and calcium antagonists.It is interesting to note the characteristic circadian variability (Fig. 24), with spasm occurring regularly at rest and early in the morning, between midnight and 5 a.m., and especially during light exercise(9).

IV. CLINICAL EXAMINATION

The clinical signs vary over time: outside the crisis, the examination may be perfectly normal, whereas in the critical phase there may be :

•A galloping rhythm and systolic murmurs associated with kinetic disorders and ischaemic mitral regurgitation.
•Hypotension
•A rapid or irregular heartbeat associated with arrhythmias (complete atrioventricular block, ventricular tachycardia and ventricular fibrillation).

A minority of patients may present with a more systemic abnormality of vasomotor tone; this may include symptoms of migraine and Raynaud's phenomenon(93).

V. ELECTROCARDIOGRAPHIC CHANGES

The ECG changes that occur during a spastic seizure include ST-segment elevation in one myocardial territory of the culprit artery, as in STEMI, indicates total occlusion of the coronary artery (Fig.25), and is generally accompanied by reciprocal ST-segment depression in the leads of the opposite territory (mirror image).
• ST-segment depression, indicating less severe myocardial ischaemia (non-transmural or subendocardial), which means that the artery is not

completely occluded, or that it receives collaterals.
- Broad, sharp or negative T waves.
- A negative U wave may also appear.

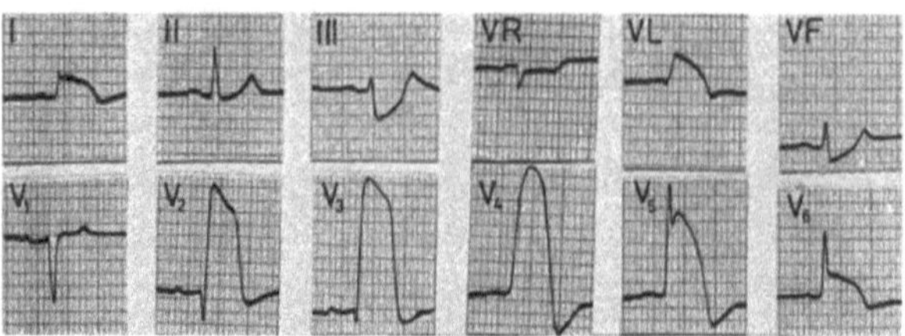

Figure 15: Surface ECG of a 65-year-old patient presenting with a Prinzmetal angina episode, with maximal ST-segment elevation in segments V1 to V6 and aVL. Coronary angiography demonstrated complete occlusion of the proximal AVI (94).

In addition to these ischaemic manifestations, various forms of arrhythmia often appear during seizures. These include ventricular arrhythmias such as ventricular extrasystoles (VSE), ventricular tachycardia and even ventricular fibrillation, bradyarrhythmias, atrioventricular block and supraventricular arrhythmias(94).

Criteria for a positive ischaemic ECG (9): If ST elevation of 0.1 mV or more, ST depression of 0.1 mV or more, or new onset of negative U waves are recorded in at least two contiguous leads on the 12-lead ECG during an attack, the ECG findings are considered indicative of an ischaemic change.

RISK AND PRECIPITATING FACTORS

I. RISK FACTORS

Hypercholesterolaemia, diabetes mellitus, hypertension, smoking and heredity are all associated with an increased risk of atherosclerotic coronary disease, but are they also responsible for the onset of coronary spasm? Researchers have been trying to answer this question for decades, and their main findings will be discussed in this chapter.

A. tobacco

In their work published in Circulation in 1993, Sugiishi et al(95) attempted to examine the risk factors for coronary vasospasm by retrospectively comparing patients with angiographically confirmed vasospastic angina and subjects with normal coronary arteries. Various risk factors were compared. The vasospasm group included 175 patients with coronary spasm, but no coronary artery narrowing exceeding 25% of the diameter. The control group comprised 176 subjects with completely normal coronary arteries and a negative response to ergonovine maleate. The odds ratio for smoking as a risk factor for vasospasm was 2.41 and (p<0.05), demonstrating that smoking appears to be a major risk factor for vasospastic angina.In some studies, the proportion of smokers among spasm patients reached 75%(96).Smoking has a significant impact on spasm in men, young subjects and the Japanese population, unlike women, older people and the Caucasian population. The substances contained in cigarettes, such as carbon monoxide and nicotine, are capable of damaging blood vessels by increasing inflammation and oxidative stress, which explains why smoking is such an important risk factor(97).

B.Hs- CRP

A link between inflammation and coronary spasm in patients with angina pectoris without coronary artery obstruction has been suspected for more than a decade. Indeed, serum high-sensitivity C-reactive protein (hs-CRP) is higher in patients with coronary spasm than in healthy individuals, suggesting that hs-CRP could be an important predictive factor.

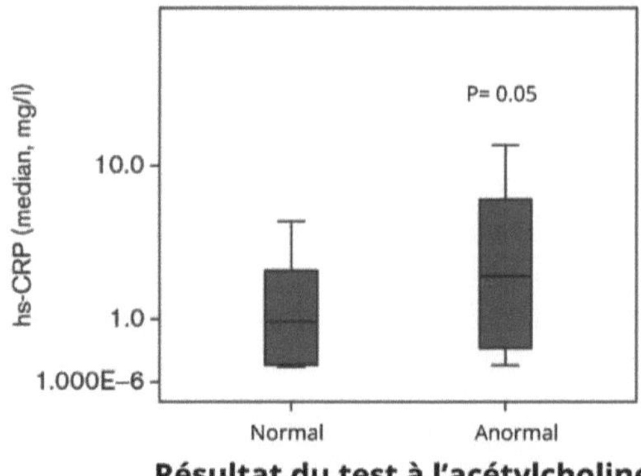

Résultat du test à l'acétylcholine

Figure 16. hs-CRP in the two groups corresponding to a normal and abnormal response to the acetylcholine test(98).

In their study and to assess whether epicardial and microvascular spasm of the coronary artery in response to acetylcholine is associated with markers of inflammation, notably Hs-CRP in patients with angina pectoris without coronary obstruction Ong et al.(98) evaluated 62 consecutive patients (26 men, age 60 ± 10 years) with angina without significant lesions on angiography (stenosis < 50%) who underwent intracoronary ACH testing to diagnose coronary spasm versus eight patients without angina who served as a control group. High-sensitivity C-reactive protein concentrations and other inflammation parameters were measured in all patients before the test.

They concluded that epicardial and microvascular coronary spasm in response to HCA correlates with concentrations were higher in patients with coronary spasm, but the result of the Mann-Whitney U test was not statistically significant [2.3 (0.4-6.7) vs. 1.0 (0,2-2,5), P = 0,05]. (Fig.26)Another study carried out by Hung et al(99) two years earlier on 897 patients came to the same conclusion, and also showed the negative prognostic value of a high HS-CRP level. (Fig.27)

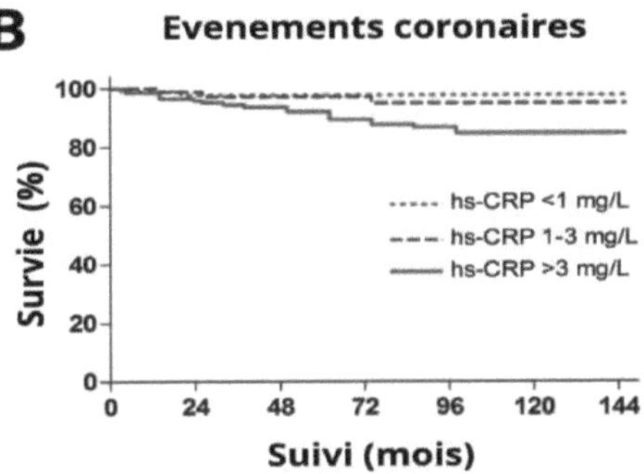

Figure 17: Prognosis of patients with coronary spasm according to hs-CRP levels (27).

C. Diabetes

Unlike coronary insufficiency of atherosclerotic origin, where diabetes is a major risk factor, the data on its relationship with coronary spasm are contradictory: for some authors, diabetes is incriminated in the genesis of spasm (79), while for others there is no statistically significant link (100,101).A rather interesting observation is that diabetes mellitus is more likely to trigger spasm in men with low Hs-CRP levels than in those with higher Hs-CRP levels(99).

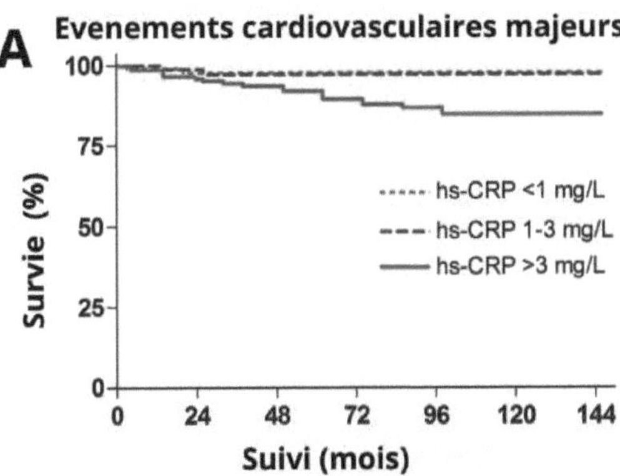

Two recently published cases of life-threatening coronary vasospasm in patients with type 2 diabetes with euglycaemic ketoacidosis induced by an SGLT2 inhibitor suggest that this drug may inhibit the activities of acetylcholine and butyrylcholine esterase, leading to reduced elimination of acetylcholine and possible induction of coronary vasospasm (102). On the other hand, in a recent cohort it was shown that spasm is a risk factor for diabetes regardless of sex. However, women under the age of 50 have a greater risk of diabetes than older women, which is not observed in men(103).

II. PRECIPITATING FACTORS

Precipitating factors may contribute to the onset of angina pectoris and act in the same patient to cause angina under different conditions.

A. Exposure to cold

Exposure to cold has been known to trigger coronary spasm since the work of Raizner et al (104) in 1980, who carried out a study on thirty-five patients undergoing coronary arteriography for the evaluation of thoracic pain syndromes and who were subjected to a cold provocation test consisting of immersing the limbs in ice-cold liquid for one minute and then undergoing coronary angiography. subsequently. Focal coronary artery spasm was induced in seven patients, ventricular ectopy and ventricular tachycardia occurred in one patient, but were readily reduced by the administration of intravenous nitroglycerin. Angiographic quantification showed that the luminal diameter of normal coronary segments decreased significantly in each group of patients in response to cold stimulation, but this response was more pronounced in the spastic angina group ($-12.7 \pm 11.5\%$ compared with control $p < 0.001$). This is explained by the reflex triggered by cold stimulation of the sympathetic nervous system.

B. Light exercise, especially early in the morning

In 1979, Yasue et al (105) demonstrated the existence of a circadian variation in exercise capacity in most patients suffering from spastic angina. They reached this conclusion by performing treadmill exercise tests early in the morning and in the afternoon of the same day in thirteen patients suffering from Prinzmetal's angina. ST-segment elevation attacks were repeatedly provoked in all 13 patients early in the morning, but in only two patients in the afternoon. However, even in the morning, moderate, single-stage exercise is more likely to induce a seizure than multi-stage exercise, which causes what is known as the "warm-up phenomenon". The possibility of inducing a seizure depends not only on the time of day, but also on the type of exercise.

C.Long-term mental stress

The effects of stress on coronary vasomotricity and blood flow have been known since the work of Yeung et al(106) in 1991 when they studied 26 patients who performed mental arithmetic under stress conditions during cardiac catheterisation with and without an acetylcholine test (four other patients who did not perform mental arithmetic served as controls). The response of the coronary arteries to mental stress varied from 38 constriction to 29% dilation, while the change in coronary blood flow varied from a 48% decrease to a 42% increase. They also found that in patients with atherosclerosis, paradoxical constriction occurs during mental stress, particularly at points of stenosis.

D.Hyperventilation

Hyperventilation is a well-known stimulus of coronary spasm - it acts by increasing arterial pH, leading to an increase in intracellular calcium influx, and may be a possible unrecognised trigger of spasm in at least some patients with variant angina(107).

E.Other

Several factors have been identified as triggers for coronary spasm:

• Magnesium deficiency(108)
• Coronary spasm itself often induces coronary spasm, creating a vicious circle.
• The catecholamines (epinephrine, norepinephrine isoproterenol, dopamine, dobutamine).
• Parasympathomimetic agents (acetylcholine, etc.).
• Anticholinesterase agents (neostigmine, etc.),
• Serotonin,
• Histamine,
• Beta-blockers,
• Withdrawal from chronic exposure to nitroglycerine,
• Cocaine,
• Alcohol: heavy alcohol consumption after stressful situations often induces coronary spasm, generally not immediately, but after several hours (109).

PATHOGENESE

The exact pathophysiology of coronary spasm is not clearly understood. However, the phenomenon is multifactorial and involves the autonomic nervous system, endothelial dysfunction, inflammation, oxidative stress, smooth muscle hyperresponsiveness, atherosclerosis, thrombosis and genetic predisposition.

I. AUTONOMIC NERVOUS SYSTEM

The relationship between spasm and the autonomic nervous system is very complicated due to the contribution of its two components: the sympathetic nervous system and the parasympathetic nervous system. In fact, the increase in parasympathetic and sympathetic tone seems to be able to induce spasm. The role of this system is supported by the frequent occurrence of spasm at midnight or at rest, i.e. when vagal activity is highest (see above), and by the ability of acetylcholine to induce ACS. Also, the increase in catecholamine levels before and after a spastic ischaemic episode and the occurrence of the latter at night during the rapid eye movement phase of sleep, marked by a reduction in vagal tone and an increase in adrenergic activity, strongly underline the contribution of the sympathetic nervous system (110,111).

II. INFLAMMATION

The relationship between inflammation and SCA was first described by Lewis et al. in a case report of spastic angina triggered by acute pericarditis leading to cardiogenic shock and death(112). Then, following the detection, in post-mortem studies, of inflammatory cells, in particular mast cells, in vasospastic coronary segments, the role of inflammation in the pathogenesis of spasm was strongly suspected(113). Fifteen years later Shimokawa et al (114) developed a porcine model of coronary spasm by applying interleukin-1□ to the coronary artery. Other studies have shown elevated levels of leukocytes and monocytes, interleukin-6 and adhesion molecules in peripheral blood (115,116). Rho-kinase activity in peripheral leukocytes independently predicts the presence and severity of vasospastic angina (117).In addition, as described above, higher levels of C-reactive protein have been reported in patients with spastic angina.

III. ENDOTHELIAL DYSFUNCTION

The coronary endothelium of a healthy subject is responsible for the production of nitric oxide, a powerful vasodilator which counterbalances the effects of vasoconstrictor metabolites, the latter of which see their activity increase in the event of endothelial dysfunction resulting in a deficiency in endogenous NO due to a dysfunction of endothelial nitric oxide synthase, this mechanism explains why several endothelium-dependent vasodilators (acetylcholine.) cause paradoxical vasoconstriction and also explains the increased efficacy of endothelium-independent vasodilators (e.g. nitrates) in this context (79,118). In a recent retrospective cohort study, concomitant endothelial dysfunction was present in the vast majority of INOCA patients with inducible coronary spasm and/or impaired adenosine-mediated vasodilation. These results indicate the importance of this phenomenon and the possible therapeutic implications (119). (Fig. 28)

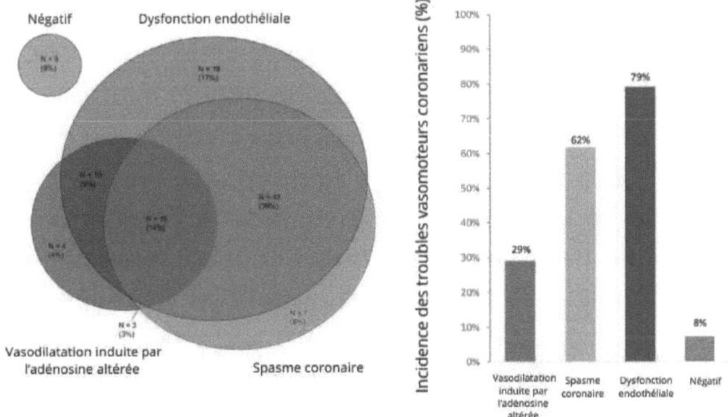

Figure 18: Incidence and overlap of coronary vasomotor disorders. (119)

IV. HYPERCONTRACTILITY OF SMOOTH MUSCLE CELLS

Relaxation and contraction of vascular smooth muscle cells are mainly regulated by dephosphorylation and phosphorylation of the myosin light chain. Rho-kinase, an enzyme present in the vascular smooth muscle cell, is a crucial regulator of hyper-contractility. It promotes contraction by directly increasing Ca2 sensitisation^{+} of the myosin light chain and indirectly increasing phosphorylation of the myosin light chain by inhibiting its binding subunit (120,121).

It has also been shown that a Rho-kinase inhibitor, hydroxyfasudil, was able to prevent coronary spasm both in the pig model and in humans (122,123) (Fig. 29).

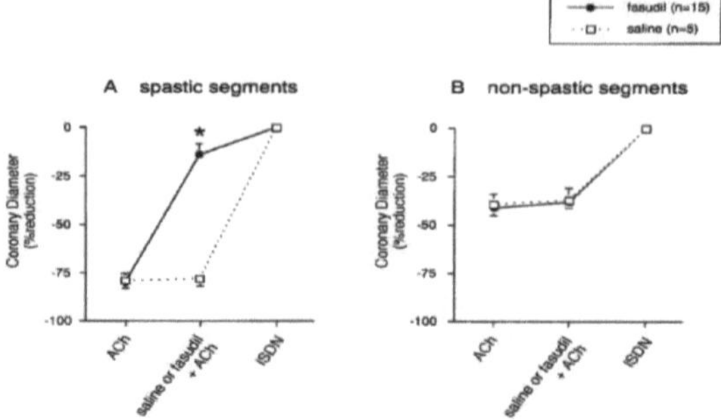

Figure 19: Changes in coronary artery diameter in spastic (A) and non-spastic (B) coronary segments in the fasudil and saline groups. *P<0.001 compared with saline group (122)

In addition, several other pathways involving nitric oxide, phospholipase C and KATP channels are also linked to the hypercontractility of vascular smooth muscle cells. In their study, Kaski et al. confirmed the hypothesis that focal spasm in patients suffering from spastic angina is mainly due to hyperreactivity of vascular smooth muscle to vasoactive stimuli, in order to investigate the relationship between local hypercontractility and endothelial dysfunction. This study showed that in these patients the ergonovine-induced spastic response was observed at the same site. This indicates that in the presence of a generalised stimulus affecting all the coronary arteries, the spasm may occur only at a site of local coronary hyperreactivity (124,125).

V. OXIDATIVE STRESS

Oxidative stress, and a disturbance in the balance between the production of reactive oxygen species represented by free radicals, such as superoxide anion and hydroxyl radicals, as well as non-radical molecules, such as hydrogen peroxide on the one hand (126)and the intracellular antioxidant defence consisting of enzymatic antioxidants (superoxide dismutase, catalase and glutathione peroxidase) and non-enzymatic antioxidants (glutathione, polyphenols and vitamins). Free radicals are metabolites that are necessary for the body to function, but their excessive production can damage cellular structures. They are characterised by the fact that they have one or more unpaired electrons. This characteristic makes them highly reactive and allows them to donate their electrons to other molecules. As a result, they lead to chain reactions and oxidative damage(127).Oxidative stress can cause vasoconstriction and endothelial damage (128), by degrading the nitric oxide released by endothelial cells, leading to microvascular dysfunction and coronary vasospasm.

VI. ATHEROSCLEROSIS AND THROMBOSIS

Atherosclerosis is characterised by the chronic accumulation of cholesterol-rich plaques and blood components in large and medium-calibre arteries, and is linked to a wide range of cardiovascular diseases. It is currently accepted that endothelial dysfunction plays a major role in the pathogenesis of atherosclerosis. Once endothelial cells have been exposed to atherogenic stresses, they become activated, which has two consequences: altered coronary vasomotricity and the expression in these cells of various adhesion molecules, such as ICAM-1, MCP-1, VCAM-1, P-selectin and E-selectin, which attract neutrophils and monocytes that subsequently penetrate the arterial wall (129). The monocytes then differentiate into macrophages in the vascular wall and engulf oxidised LDL to become foam cells, which constitute the basic histopathological lesion of atherosclerosis(130). Recently, a number of studies have shown correlations between atherosclerosis and vasomotor dysfunction, and this relationship is a two-way street, with spasm occurring more frequently in arteries with atherosclerotic segments(127) ; in 1994 Yamagishi et al. used intracoronary imaging in a study of twenty-two patients suffering from chest pain at rest or during exercise, or both, who have vasospasm triggered by intracoronary administration of ergonovine maleate that atherosclerosis is present at the site of focal vasospasm, even in the absence of angiographically significant coronary disease(131). (Fig.30) On the other hand, Pelligrini et al. found that patients with spasm had more advanced atherosclerosis and a higher prevalence of vulnerable plaques, larger lipid bodies and neovascularisation than those without vasomotor problems(132).

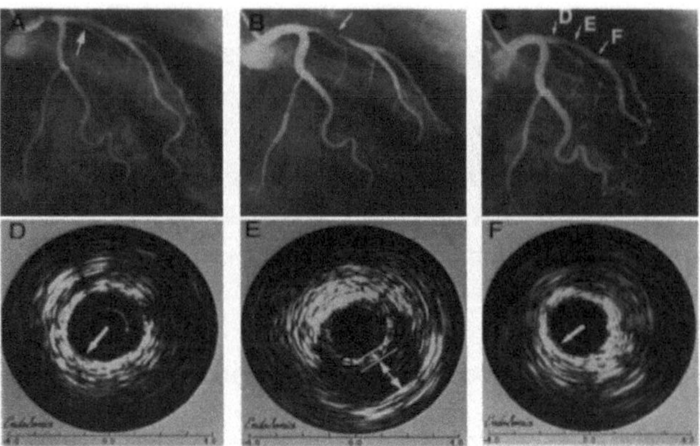

Figure 20: Angiographic and intravascular ultrasound findings in the patient with focal vasospasm of the LAI: A, Prior to ergonovine administration, there were minor luminal irregularities in the coronary artery (arrow). B, 2.5 minutes after intracoronary administration of ergonovine (0.01 mg), this segment was severely narrowed to 99% stenosis (arrow). C, Intracoronary administration of nitroglycerin (0.25 mg) relieved the narrowing and irregularities of the lumen remained at the site of spasm (arrow). D, The intravascular ultrasound image at the proximal site of vasospasm (arrow D in C) shows a thin intimal leading edge and a thin echogenic zone (arrow). E, At the site of vasospasm (arrow E in C), there was a thickened intimal leading edge (arrow) and a thickened echogenic zone representing a non-circumferential atherosclerotic lesion of I to 8 hours. F, The distal site of vasospasm (arrow F in C) showed no evidence of atherosclerosis (131).

In addition, numerous studies have shown that the presence of atherosclerosis with spasm is associated with poorer patient outcomes, such as the work of Shin et al. which looked at 2,129 patients from the VA-KOREA (Vasospastic Angina in Korea) registry(133).It should also be mentioned that spasm could destabilise a plaque, leading to coronary thrombosis and myocardial infarction(134).Oshima et al. in 1990 in their work on the relationship between spasm and coagulation found that plasma levels of fibrinopeptide A, a marker of thrombin generation, are increased after spastic attacks, something which is not seen in exertional angina (135) and Ogawa et al.(136) were able to demonstrate a circadian variation in levels parallel to that of attacks (Fig.31). Similar results for platelet activation have also been noted (137). These results indicate that spasm can trigger coronary thrombosis and may play an important role in the pathogenesis of acute coronary syndromes.

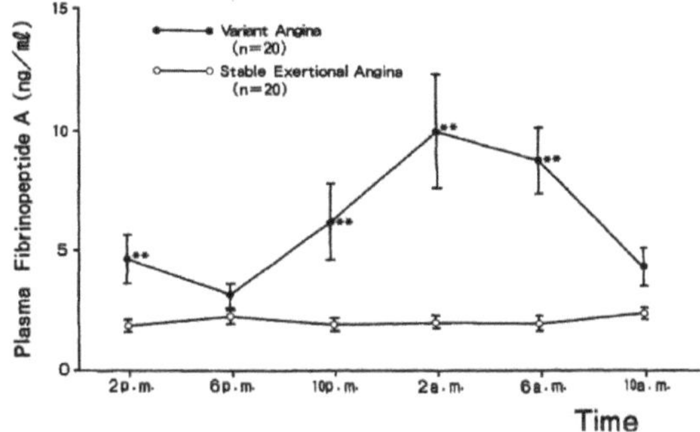

Figure 21: Line graph showing plasma fibrinopeptide A levels (ng/ml) in patients with variant angina and stable stress angina. (p<0.01)(136)

VII. MAGNESIUM

Magnesium is considered to be an endogenous calcium antagonist, and magnesium infusion suppresses the hyperventilation-induced crisis in patients with coronary spasm(108). Magnesium deficiency exists in 45% of patients with variant angina and may be linked to the genesis of coronary spasm in some of these patients(138).

VIII. GENETICS

Studies on genetic mutations or polymorphisms in the pathogenesis of coronary spasm have been contradictory. It has been shown that mutations or polymorphisms in the endothelial NO synthase gene and polymorphisms in the paraoxonase I gene are significantly associated with spasm. The other genes involved code for :

• Adrenergic and serotonin receptors,
• Angiotensin-converting enzyme,
• Inflammatory cytokines,
• NADH/NADPH oxidase in men,
• ALDH (aldehyde dehydrogenase) activity: ALDH2 deficiency, which is more common in the East Asian population, is strongly associated, with an increased effect due to the co-existence of smoking and/or alcohol (79,139).

IX. SPECIAL CASE OF KOUNIS SYNDROME

Kounis syndrome is an unfamiliar form of vasospastic angina occurring in a hypersensitive situation. It is known as "allergic angina" or "allergic myocardial infarction" (140). Type 1 is a pure spasm involving a normal coronary artery, while type 2 is a spasm occurring in an atherosclerotic coronary artery causing plaque rupture. Various inflammatory mediators such as histamines and leukotrienes massively secreted into the peripheral circulation during a hypersensitivity reaction trigger the spasm through their effects on the smooth muscle of the coronary vessels.

DIAGNOSTIC

The diagnosis of coronary spasm depends first and foremost on the semiological analysis of the clinical presentation (type of pain and its characteristics, triggering factors, etc.), as well as the cardiovascular clinical examination and the ECG (see chapter on clinical characteristics). However, we must not lose sight of the fact that this clinical analysis is highly inadequate and not very discriminating, and we must not forget that the key element here is the spasm, which must be visualised by angiography, either spontaneously or induced by medication.

The diagnosis is based on the following three considerations:

• Typical clinical presentation,
• Evidence of transient ischaemia on the ECG during the angina episode,
• Demonstration of spontaneous or induced coronary vasospasm.

Before turning to angiography and provocation tests, we review the usefulness of other non-invasive tests.

I. HOLTER RECORDING ECG

In patients with vasospastic angina, chest pain occurs in approximately 20-30% of episodes of ST-segment ischaemic change, and many episodes of coronary spasm are asymptomatic(9). Because seizures occur frequently between night and early morning at rest, ischaemic ST-segment changes that occur during a seizure often cannot be recorded, except in the context of hospitalisation. In such cases, Holter recording is the most useful test. If ischaemia persists for 5 minutes or more, chest pain is likely to be present; ECG recordings during symptomatic ischaemic episodes should be assessed in detail for ST segment level characteristics and the occurrence of arrhythmia. Attention should also be paid to asymptomatic ST-T segment changes.

II. TEST EFFORT

Stress testing is not recommended, especially in patients whose condition is unstable and in whom acute coronary syndrome cannot be ruled out (**Class III**). It may be considered in **class IIb** in patients whose condition is stable(9).

If an early morning exercise test reveals at least one of the following, and the ECG and exercise tolerance results in the morning differ from those during the day, the patient may be suffering from vasospastic angina:

•Appearance of ST-segment elevation of 0.1 mV or more in at least two contiguous leads during the stress test.
•Appearance of ST-segment depression of 0.1 mV or more in at least two contiguous leads during the stress test.
•Appearance o f negative U waves not observed at rest during the stress test.

III. MYOCARDIAL SCINTIGRAPHY

As with stress testing, myocardial scintigraphy is not recommended in unstable patients, but it may be considered in class IIb in stable patients, and if performed with I metaiodobenzylguanidine (I MIBG), according to Sakata et al. it can identify high-risk patients, even among those with spastic angina who were previously considered low risk(141).

IV. HYPERVENTILATION TEST

This test is preferably performed at rest, early in the morning, after an interval of at least 48 hours following the administration of vasoactive drugs. The patient is placed in the supine position, the 12-lead ECG and resting blood pressure are taken, and then the patient is asked to hyperventilate vigorously (goal: respiratory rate of 25 times/minute or more) for 6 minutes, whenever possible. The 12-lead ECG should be monitored during this stage and for the next 10 minutes, and blood pressure should be taken every minute. If an anginal attack occurs or there is a significant change in the ST-T segment on the ECG

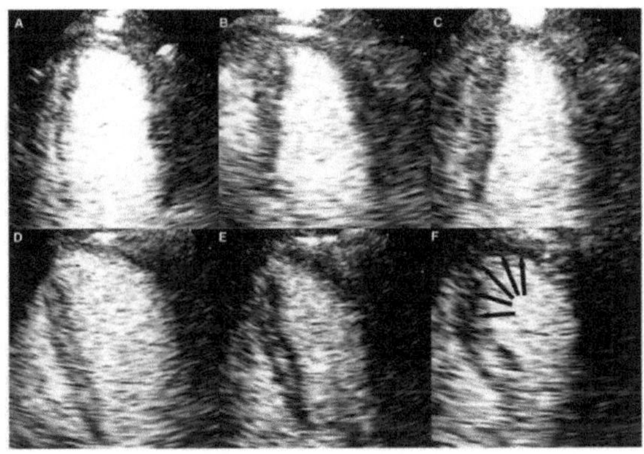

Figure 22: Myocardial contrast echocardiography. The top row shows normal left ventricular diastolic (A) and systolic (B) cavity size at baseline and normal myocardial perfusion (C). The bottom row shows the corresponding diastolic (D) and systolic (E) images after intracoronary injection of 200-µg acetylcholine, showing a dilated cavity in systole compared with rest and clear perfusion defects (F, arrows). (142) during artificial hyperventilation, this should be stopped immediately and a fast-acting nitrate administered immediately.

The hyperventilation test is positive if at least one of the following findings is obtained:

•Appearance of ST-segment elevation of 0.1 mV or more in at least two contiguous leads during the hyperventilation test.
•Appearance of ST-segment depression of 0.1 mV or more in at least two contiguous leads during the hyperventilation test.
•Appearance o f negative U waves not observed at rest during the hyperventilation test

It should be noted that this test is indicated in class IIa for patients suspected of suffering from vasospastic angina with a low frequency of attacks and in class IIb for patients suspected of suffering from vasospastic angina with a high frequency of attacks(9).

V.THE TOMOGRAPHY BY EMISSION (PET SCAN)

It is a well-validated technique that can not only help assess coronary vasomotor function by providing non-invasive, accurate and reproducible quantification of myocardial blood flow and coronary flow reserve in humans, but also help reveal the tissue image of coronary spasm. In addition to its high cost, it could also be useful for assessing coronary artery function and inflammation of the perivascular tissue surrounding these arteries (96,142).

VI. ECHOCARDIOGRAPHY MYOCARDIAC FROM CONTRAST

Ong et al(143) published a clinical case of transient myocardial ischaemia by contrast echocardiography during Ach-induced vasospastic angina (Fig.32).This non-invasive technique is capable of providing indirect functional information on the microcirculation and thus helps to diagnose spastic angina. However, it still has a number of limitations due to the technical difficulties involved in performing it and the biases involved in interpreting it. Few of the available studies have focused on coronary spasm.

VII.ANGIOGRAPHY

Coronary angiography may reveal focal or diffuse spasm of one or more coronary arteries (Fig.33); associated with typical symptoms, ECG changes or even ventricular dysfunction, this spasm may be pathognomonic of the condition. Most patients with variant angina and proven coronary vasospasm have angiographic evidence of atherosclerotic coronary artery disease, usually mild. Focal spasm most often occurs within 1 cm of an angiographically apparent obstruction. If minimal or no angiographic signs of coronary artery disease are found in a patient who has recently presented with angina at rest with transient ST-segment elevation within the INOCA framework, the most likely diagnosis is that of variant angina.

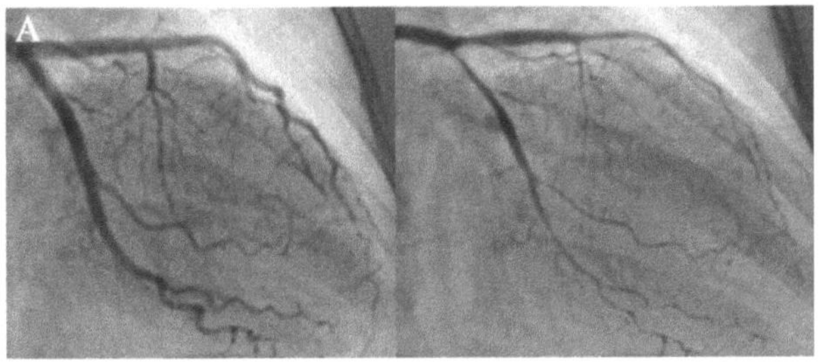

Figure 23: Ach-induced spasm of the IVA and circumflex (96)

VIII. CHALLENGE TESTS

Spasm provocation tests involve the administration of a provocative stimulus (usually intracoronary acetylcholine, but intracoronary or intravenous ergonovine may also be used) during invasive coronary angiography, with monitoring of the patient's symptoms, ECG and angiography. A positive challenge test for coronary artery spasm should induce all of the following:

• Reproduction of the usual chest pain,

• Ischaemic ECG changes

• Vasoconstriction > 90% on angiography, which has been considered since the COVADIS symposium consensus as the angiographic threshold for diagnosing inducible spasm.

If this vasoconstriction occurs within the limits of an isolated coronary segment, it is termed focal spasm, whereas when it affects 2 or more adjacent coronary segments, it is termed diffuse spasm(144).The test result is considered equivocal if the provocative stimulus does not induce the three components.Validation studies have demonstrated high sensitivity and specificity for ergonovine (91% and 97%, respectively) and acetylcholine (90% and 99%, respectively) protocols in the diagnosis of spontaneous spasm(145).

A. Risks

Unlike invasive challenge tests, which allow rapid detection and treatment of induced spasm, non-invasive bedside challenge testing has been associated with significant adverse events, including death, as detection and treatment of induced spasm is delayed. It is currently accepted that the risk profile of invasive testing is similar to that of other invasive coronary procedures, although there is a 6.8% incidence of cardiac arrhythmias(145).

B. Indications

Given the risks associated with provocative spasm testing, the procedure should be performed by experienced personnel in patients whose risks and benefits have been carefully assessed (145):

Class I

•Suspected history of spastic angina without a documented episode, particularly if :
•Resting angina in response to nitrates, and/or
•Marked diurnal variation in onset of symptoms/exercise tolerance, and/or
•Resting angina without obstructive coronary disease
•Does not respond to empirical treatment
•Acute coronary syndrome in the absence of a culprit lesion
•Unexplained cardiac arrest revived
•Unexplained syncope with a history of chest pain
•Recurrent rest angina after angiographically successful angioplasty

Class IIa

•Invasive tests for patients diagnosed non-invasively and not responding to drug treatment
•,documented spontaneous episode of spastic angina to determine the "site and mode" of the spasm

Class IIb

•Invasive tests for patients diagnosed non-invasively and responding to drug treatment

Class III

•Current acute coronary syndrome
•Severe multitruncal coronary disease, including TCG stenosis

•Severe myocardial dysfunction (class IIb if symptoms suggest vasospasm)

•Patients with no symptoms suggestive of spastic angina.

IX. IMAGING INTRACORONARY

Intracoronary imaging using intravascular ultrasound (IVUS) and optical coherence tomography (OCT) is playing an emerging but limited role in the assessment of coronary spasm. IVUS can identify the

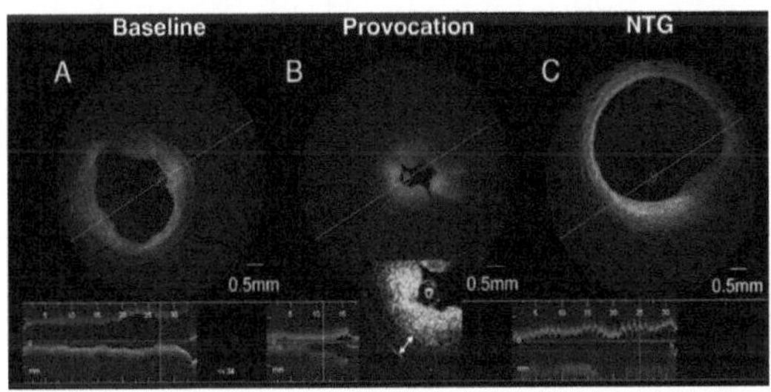

Figure 24: Representative optical coherence tomography (OCT) images of a spasm lesion (A, B, C)

NTG = nitroglycerine (146)

plaque composition and intimal hyperplasia at the site of focal spasm in the absence of significant angiographic disease. In parallel, OCT can accurately delineate structural changes in spasmodic coronary arteries. Characteristic abnormalities in these patients include the presence of an intimal bulge and thickening of the media during spasm; these abnormalities disappear after administration of nitroglycerin (146,147).(Fig.34) The following table summarises the diagnostic criteria established by the Coronary Vasomotor Disorders International Study Group (COVADIS) (145,87)

Elements of the diagnostic criteria for vasospastic angina :

{1} Nitrate-responsive angina during a spontaneous episode, with at least one of the following:

• Resting angina, especially between night and early morning
• Marked diurnal variation in exercise tolerance - reduced in the morning
• Hyperventilation can precipitate an episode

- Calcium channel blockers {but not b-blockers} suppress the episodes
{2} Transient ischaemic ECG changes during a spontaneous episode, including any of the following in at least two contiguous leads:
- ST segment elevation;? 0. 1 mV
- ST segment depression; ? 0.1 mV
- New negative U waves

{3} Coronary artery spasm defined as transient total or subtotal occlusion of the coronary artery {.90% constriction} with angina and ischaemic ECG changes either spontaneously or in response to a provocative stimulus {typically acetylcholine, ergot or hyperventilation}.

TREATMENT

The optimal management of vasospastic angina includes lifestyle modifications, conventional pharmacotherapy, and cardiac interventions for well-selected clinical subgroups.

I. CHANGES TO THE LIFE MOSDE

Given that endothelial dysfunction is an important element in the genesis of the disease, the elimination or control of factors likely to alter endothelial function or increase oxidative stress is essential:

A. Stop smoking

Cigarette smoking is an important risk factor in coronary spasm, and is also one of the most important risk factors for atherosclerosis. In a 2016 study, Choi et al. demonstrated the negative impact of smoking on the prognosis of patients with coronary vasospasm, finding that the cigarette-smoking coronary spasm group had a higher incidence of recurrent angina during the 3-year clinical follow-up compared with the non-smoking group. They concluded that smoking cessation, combined with intensive medical treatment and close clinical follow-up, can help prevent recurrent angina(148). (Fig.35)

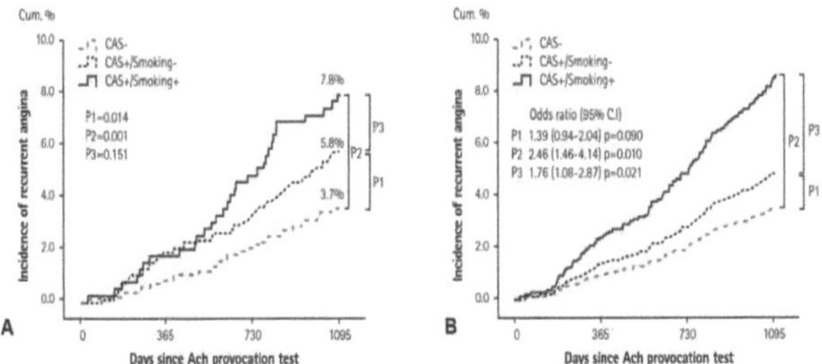

Figure 25: Survival curve analysis describing the cumulative incidence of recurrent angina at 3 years (148)

CAS-: group of patients without coronary artery spasm, CAS+/Sm-: group of non-smoking patients with CAS, CAS+/Sm+: group of smoking patients with CAS.

B. Controlling risk factors cardiovascular

The elimination or control of all risk factors for coronary atherosclerosis is also necessary in the case of coronary spasm:

- Blood pressure control
- Maintaining your ideal body weight
- Correction of glucose intolerance
- Correction of lipid abnormalities
- Avoid excessive fatigue, as strenuous exercise during the day can trigger attacks in the middle of the night or in the early hours of the morning.
- Avoid mental or emotional stress, which is a very important substrate for seizures, and anger or fear can induce seizures.
- Stop drinking alcohol, which can induce coronary spasm attacks several hours after consumption in susceptible patients, particularly those with the aldehyde dehydrogenase polymorphism (ALDH2)(149).

C. Avoiding precipitating factors or

- Hyperventilation and exposure to cold should be avoided.
- Drugs that may induce coronary spasm should be avoided. These include catecholamines, muscarinic agonists, ergot alkaloids, prostaglandins, alcohol and propranolol.
- Magnesium deficiency must be treated promptly by supplementation.
- Certain substances should be avoided: catecholamines, cholinergic agents, serotonergic agents, beta-blockers, CNS stimulants, general anaesthesia.

II. MEDICAL TREATMENT

A. Nitro derivatives

Nitrates are converted in vivo to NO, and the coronary arteries involved in the spasm are very sensitive to nitrates. An attack of coronary spasm can generally be rapidly relieved by sublingual administration or oral spraying of nitroglycerin or dinitrate. isosorbide. In the event of refractory spasm, intravenous or intracoronary injection of these drugs may be necessary. The administration of long-acting nitrates for the prevention of coronary spasm is also recommended, but it should be borne in mind that the efficacy of nitrates is reduced by the phenomenon of tolerance. In clinical practice, intermittent treatment with a nitrate-free window of at least 8 hours has been recommended.

B. Calcium channel blockers

Calcium channel blockers (CCBs), which suppress the entry of Ca^{2+} into vascular smooth muscle cells, are highly effective in preventing coronary artery spasm and are considered to be drugs of first choice for the treatment of vasospastic angina. They can be used safely, without adverse effects, at the usual doses. The efficacy of these drugs in treating coronary spasm is often spectacular, and overall, 40% of patients will no longer suffer from angina pectoris thanks to calcium antagonists. It should be noted that the timing of administration of these drugs is important, as attacks of coronary spasm generally occur between midnight and early morning. These drugs should therefore be administered before going to bed. Doses should also be increased gradually for each patient, taking account of side effects. Non-dihydropyridines (DHP) are the preferred first-line agent, while a combination of non-DHP and DHP is recommended for persistent symptoms. Moderate to high doses are often required, e.g. verapamil 240-480 mg daily, diltiazem 180-540 mg daily, nifedipine 60-120 mg daily.

C. Other

Magnesium, statins, antioxidants such as vitamin C and E, converting enzyme inhibitors, angiotensin II receptor antagonists, anti-inflammatory agents such as aspirin, or oestrogens in postmenopausal women, can also have beneficial effects on coronary spasm. Nicorandil, the RoK inhibitor and fasudil are all second-line alternatives(87).

III. INTERVENTIONAL TREATMENT

A. Coronary angioplasty

Percutaneous coronary intervention is not generally recommended, as the spasm is likely to recur outside the stented segment. However, in certain patients with focal damage refractory to medical treatment, angioplasty may be reasonable(150).

B. The sympathectomy,

It involves the removal of T2-T4 sympathetic ganglia, reduced angina in a small study by lin et al who compared the clinical results of sympathectomy with those of conventional treatment in 79 patients with refractory spastic angina(151); however, there was no angiographic reassessment to determine whether the vasoconstriction had been resolved.

C. Implantable defibrillator

In patients who have suffered ventricular arrhythmias or cardiac arrest following coronary spasm, recurrent arrhythmias may occur, even with medical treatment tolerated to the maximum. The role of implantable defibrillators, in addition to medical treatment in these conditions, is still debated but is often recommended on the basis of these data. They are not recommended in cases of spasm without documented ventricular arrhythmia/cardiac arrest.

IV. TREATMENT SURGERY

Both coronary artery bypass grafting and angioplasty can be considered for patients with significant epicardial stenosis. The success of these procedures is greater in patients with focal, non-diffuse atherosclerotic stenosis.

PRONOSTIC

The natural history of variant angina or coronary spasm is generally characterised by periods of recurrent attacks of varying duration alternating with periods when the patient is asymptomatic. Long-term survival is generally good, provided patients follow a healthy lifestyle and take their medication. Factors predictive of a poor prognosis include the presence of organic coronary disease, acute coronary syndrome or arrhythmia. Advanced age, multi-vessel spasm, high hsCRP and out-of-hospital cardiac arrest are other significant predictors of mortality(152,153).Waters et al. demonstrated a survival rate of 95%, 90% and 87% at 1, 2 and 3 years respectively(154). (Fig. 36) Spontaneous remission can be observed without medical treatment in 30% of cases, but long-term maintenance of calcium antagonists is generally recommended to reduce the future risk of arrhythmia or myocardial infarction.

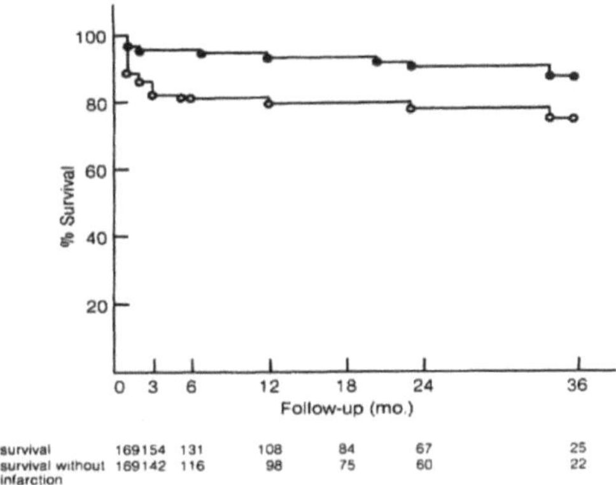

Figure 26: Survival and survival without myocardial infarction

CASE CLINICAL

I. CASE PRESENTATION

A 53-year-old overweight woman (BMI: 28) with a history of hypertension on Candesartan 16 mg presented to the emergency department with chest pain that had been severe for 3 hours. The ECG showed ST-segment elevation in the inferior leads and ST-segment depression in the aVL leads (Fig. 37).

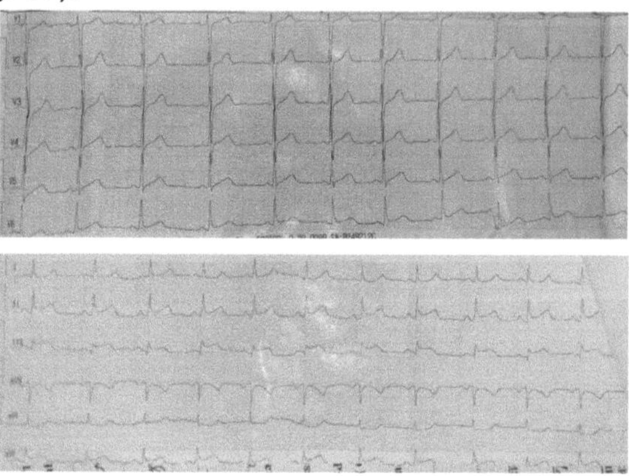

Figure 27: ECG showing ST elevation in the inferior leads

On arrival at A&E, the patient was haemodynamically stable, with an elevated blood pressure of 145/90 mmHg and a heart rate of 70 beats per minute, and was still complaining of excruciating and persistent pain. Laboratory tests revealed blood glucose of 1.3 g/l, creatinine of 7 mg/dl and urea of 0.20 g/l. Troponin I levels were high, at 0.86 ng/ml. Aspirin was administered (loading dose of 250 mg po) with a loading dose of clopedogrel (300 mg po), and LMWH, then she was transferred to the catheterisation room for primary angioplasty. Coronary angiography showed tight stenosis of the distal interventricular artery, a healthy circumflex and tight stenosis of the right coronary artery at the level of the $3^{\text{ième}}$ segment, as well as occlusion of the PVI (culprit artery) (see Figures 38, 39 and 40 below).

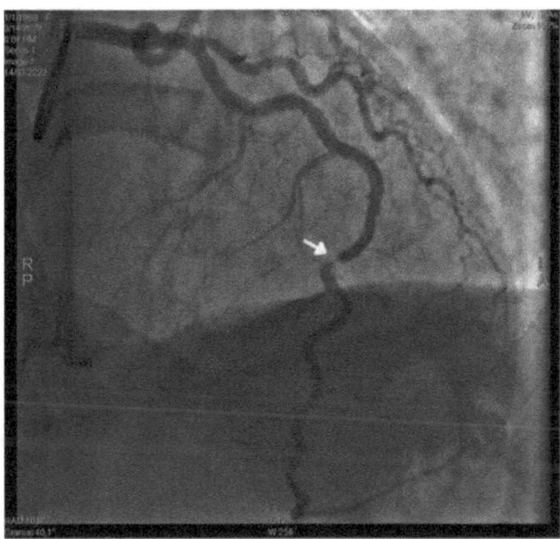

Figure 28: Cranial right anterior oblique view showing distal stenosis of the VIA (arrow)

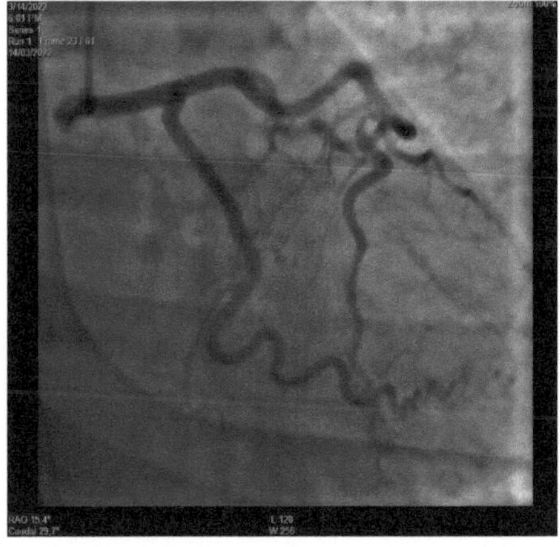

Right anterior caudal oblique view showing a healthy circumflex

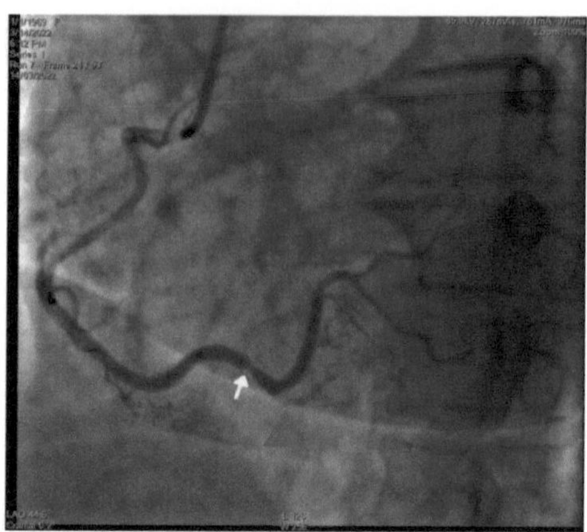

Figure 30: Left anterior oblique view showing stenosis of segment III of the CD (arrow) and occlusion of the ostium of the IVP (red triangle).

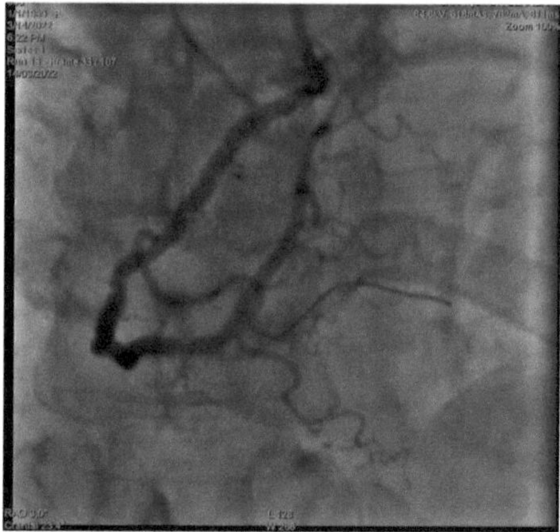

Figure 29: The IVP is always occluded after thrombo-aspiration

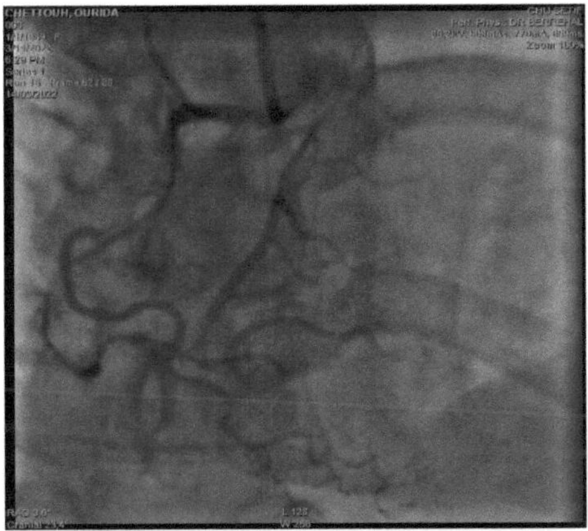

Figure 32: Diffuse CD spasm

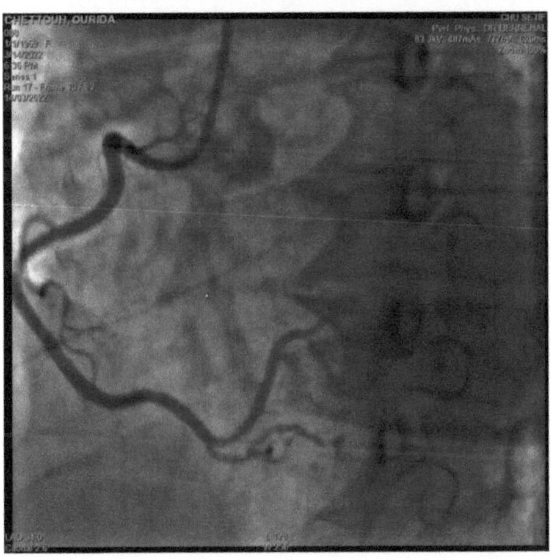

Figure 31: almost complete disappearance of lesions

A 0.014 guide wire of 1ère intention was inserted distal to the posterior interventricular, and thromboaspiration was performed without success (Fig.40). The patient then suddenly presented with worsening chest pain which became unbearable, she became agitated and had a vagal malaise, an injection of contrast product to assess the situation objectiveed a diffuse spasm of the entire coronary tree (Fig.41). At this point we realised that we were dealing with ACS due to coronary spasm, and a bolus of 1 mg nicardipine and 1.5 mg trinitrin was immediately administered intracoronary, resulting in a marked clinical improvement.

Angiographic examination showed that the spasm had disappeared and the PVI had reopened. (Fig.42)We recommended that the patient be put on calcium antagonists: Tildiem 180 mg per day in combination with molsidomine 12 mg per day.Progress was favourable with no recurrence of angina, left ventricular function was restored, and there was only hypokinesia of the inferior wall. An angiographic check after seven days showed complete disappearance of all lesions, including the VIA. (Fig.43, 44)

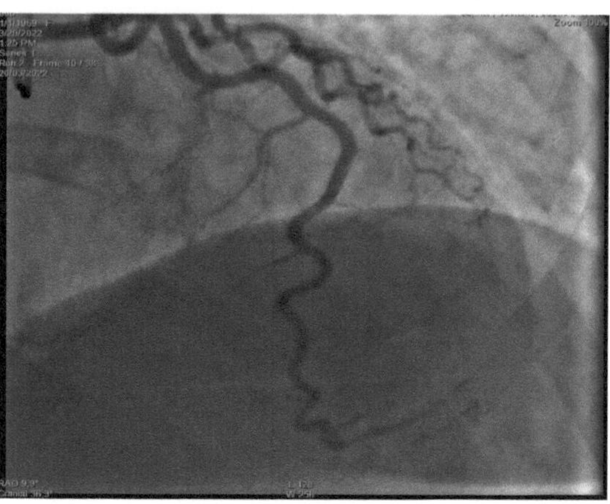

Figure 33: Angiographic control showing complete disappearance of the VIA lesion.

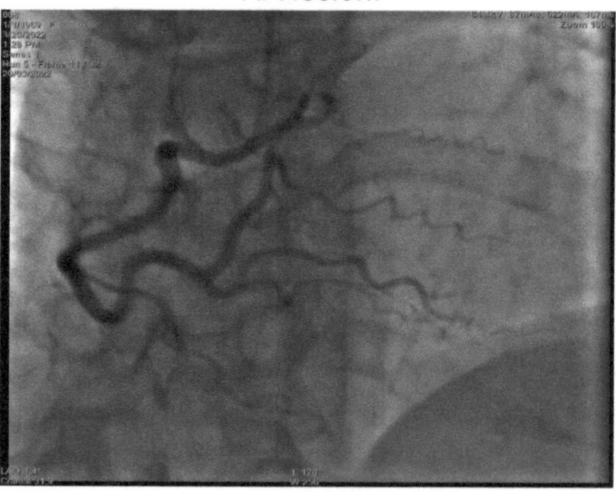

Figure 34: Angiogram showing complete disappearance of CD lesions.

II. DISCUSSION

This case provides a good illustration of the importance and seriousness of coronary spasm. The reduction in calibre caused an imbalance between O2 supply and demand, which was very severe, leading to myocardial ischaemia. An important fact to be added to this context is that this spasm was prolonged over time (more than 3 hours) and was therefore expressed as a STEMI.This case also illustrates a very interesting fact: the difficulty of making a positive diagnosis. Remember that our initial strategy was thromboaspiration, thinking that it was atherothrombosis, and that the true diagnosis was atherothrombosis. was only introduced by chance when the spasm worsened before our very eyes.Finally, it is worth highlighting the contrast between the severity of the clinical presentation and the potential risks, and the simplicity of the treatment.

CONCLUSION

The coronary arteries have vasomotor properties that enable them to regulate blood flow, so coronary constriction is not always pathological. Nevertheless, in certain situations, it becomes more predominant, leading to a wide range of clinical symptoms, from angina to acute coronary syndrome and sudden cardiac death, which can be the revelatory event.Vasospastic angina is an underestimated cause of chest pain. An important but often overlooked factor, it is a complex multifactorial disease that can lead to serious complications.
Endothelial dysfunction, hypercontractility of vascular smooth muscle cells and the predominance of vasoconstrictive metabolites characterise its complex pathogenesis. Furthermore, the most recent discoveries have shown that inflammation plays an essential role in modulating all its stages. The important role of atherosclerosis and thrombosis has also been highlighted.Early diagnosis is essential, and involves a traditional clinical approach, ECG and angiography, with the use of invasive pharmacological provocation tests, which remain the cornerstone of the diagnosis. Medical imaging, particularly endocoronary imaging, contrast echography and PET scans, are in full development and may become key players in the near future.Lifestyle modifications, smoking abstinence and conventional pharmacotherapy with optimal dosing of calcium antagonists are the mainstays of current management, although the treatment of refractory cases remains an ongoing challenge. Given that recurrent episodes of angina pectoris are frequently observed, it is essential to continue studies in order to better define the molecular pathways responsible and develop more effective treatments for vasospastic angina.

BIBLIOGRAPHY

1. Thygesen K, Alpert JS, Jaffe AS, Chaitman BR, Bax JJ, Morrow DA, et al. Fourth universal definition of myocardial infarction (2018). European Heart Journal. 14 Jan 2019;40(3):237-69.

2. William Osler,. The Lumleian Lectures ON ANGINA PECTORIS. The Lancet. 1910;175(4517):839-44.

3. Wilson, Frank N, Johnston, Franklin D. The occurrence in angina pectoris of electrocardiographic changes similar in magnitude and in kind to those produced by myocardial infarction. American Heart Journal. 22(1):64-74.

4. PRINZMETAL M, KENNAMER R, MERLISS R, WADA T, BOR N. Angina
pectoris. I. A variant form of angina pectoris; preliminary report. The American Journal of Medicine. Sept 1959;27(3):375-88.

5. Maseri A, Severi S, L'Abbate A, Chierchia S, Marzilli M, Ballestra AM, et al. "Variant" Angina: One Aspect of a Continuous Spectrum of Vasospastic Myocardial Ischemia. 1978;42.

6. Brown BG. Observations Linking the Clinical Spectrum of Ischemic Heart Disease to the Dynamic Pathology of Coronary Atherosclerosis. ARCH INTERN MED. May 1981;141.

7. Bugiardini R, Pozzati A, Ottani F, Morgagni GL, Puddu P. Vasotonic angina: A spectrum of ischemic syndromes involving function abnormalities of the epicardial and microvascular coronary circulation. Journal of the American College of Cardiology. August 1993;22(2):417-25.

8. Bugiardini R, Cenko E. A Short History of Vasospastic Angina. Journal of the American College of Cardiology. nov 2017;70(19):2359-62.
9. JCS Joint Working Group. Guidelines for Diagnosis and Treatment of Patients With Vasospastic Angina (Coronary Spastic Angina) (JCS 2013):- Digest Version -. Circ J. 2014;78(11):2779-801.

10. Joshi SD, Joshi SS, Athavale SA. Origins of the Coronary Arteries

and Their Significance. Clinics. Jan 2010;65(1):79-84.

11. Nornina Anatomica 1989 6th edition. Edinburgh: (:hurchill 1,ivingstone.

12. Turner K, Navaratnam V. The positions of coronary arterial ostia. Clin Anat. 1996;9(6):376-80.

13. Waller BF, Orr CM, Slack JD, Pinkerton CA, Van Tassel J, Peters T. Anatomy, histology, and pathology of coronary arteries: A review relevant to new interventional and imaging techniques-Part I. Clin Cardiol. June 1992;15(6):451-7.

14. Roberts WC. Major anomalies of coronary arterial origin seen in adulthood. American Heart Journal. May 1986;111(5):941-63.

15. Muriago M, Sheppard MN, Yen Ho S, Anderson RH. Location of the coronary arterial orifices in the normal heart. Clin Anat. 1997;10(5):297-302.

16. Left Coronary Artery I Atlas of Human Cardiac Anatomy [Internet]. [cited 25 Jan.2024].Available from at: https://www.vhlab.umn.edu/atlas/coronary-arteries/left-coronary-artery/index.shtml

17. Kenhub [Internet]. [cited 25 Jan 2024]. Left coronary artery. Available from: https://www.kenhub.com/en/library/anatomy/left-coronary-artery

18. Iaizzo PA, editor. Handbook of cardiac anatomy, physiology, and devices. Totowa, N.J: Humana Press; 2005. 469 p. (Current clinical oncology).

19. Anatomy_ A Regional Atlas of the Human Body.pdf.

20. Shriki JE, Shinbane JS, Rashid MA, Hindoyan A, Withey JG, DeFrance A, et al. Identifying, characterizing, and classifying congenital anomalies of the coronary arteries. Radiographics. 2012;32(2):453-68.

21. Gartner LP. Color atlas and text of histology. Seventh edition. Philadelphia: Wolters Kluwer; 2018. 599 p.

22. Michael H. Ross, Wojciech Pawlina. histology a text and atlas with correlated cell and molecular biology. 7th edition. Lippincott Williams &

Wilkins; 2015. 984 pages.

23. Mescher AL, Junqueira LCU. Junqueira's basic histology: text and atlas. Fourteenth edition. New York: Mcgraw-Hill Education; 2016.

24. Deussen A, Ohanyan V, Jannasch A, Yin L, Chilian W. Mechanisms of metabolic coronary flow regulation. Journal of Molecular and Cellular Cardiology. Apr 2012;52(4):794-801.

25. Brooks H, Kirk ES, Vokonas PS, Urschel CW, Sonnenblick EH. Performance of the right ventricle under stress: relation to right coronary flow. J Clin Invest. 1 Oct 1971;50(10):2176-83.

26. Heward SJ, Widrich J. Coronary Perfusion Pressure. In: StatPearls [Internet]. Treasure Island (FL): StatPearls Publishing; 2024 [cited 2024 Jan 30]. Available from: http://www.ncbi.nlm.nih.gov/books/NBK551531/

27. Duncker DJ, Bache RJ. Regulation of Coronary Blood Flow During Exercise. Physiological Reviews. July 2008;88(3):1009-86.

28. Nguyen T, Do H, Pham T, Vu LT, Zuin M, Rigatelli G. Left ventricular dysfunction causing ischemia in patients with patent coronary arteries. Perfusion. march 2018;33(2):115-22.

29. Johnson PC. REVIEW OF PREVIOUS STUDIES AND CURRENT THEORIES OF AUTOREGULATION. Circ Res. August 1964;15:SUPPL:2-9.

30. Feigl EO. Coronary autoregulation. J Hypertens Suppl. Sept 1989;7(4):S55-58; discussion S59.

31. Bayliss WM. On the local reactions of the arterial wall to changes of internal pressure. The Journal of Physiology. May 28, 1902;28(3):220-31.

32. Davis MJ, Sikes PJ. Myogenic responses of isolated arterioles: test for a rate-sensitive mechanism. American Journal of Physiology-Heart and Circulatory Physiology. 1 Dec 1990;259(6):H1890-900.

33. Davis MJ, Hill MA. Signaling Mechanisms Underlying the Vascular Myogenic Response. Physiological Reviews. 1 Apr 1999;79(2):387-423.

34. Goodwill AG, Dick GM, Kiel AM, Tune JD. Regulation of Coronary

Blood Flow. In: Terjung R, editor. Comprehensive Physiology [Internet]. 1re ed. Wiley; 2017 [cited Feb 8, 2024]. p. 321-82. Available from: https://onlinelibrary.wiley.com/doi/10.1002/cphy.c160016

35. Woollard HH. THE INNERVATION OF THE HEART.

36. Malor R, Griffin CJ, Taylor S. Innervation of the blood vessels in guinea-pig atria. Cardiovascular Research. 1 Jan 1973;7(1):95-104.

37. Lever JD, Ahmed M, Irvine G. Neuromuscular and intercellular relationships in the coronary arterioles. A morphological and quantitative study by light and electron microscopy.

38. Ito M, Zipes DP. Efferent sympathetic and vagal innervation of the canine right ventricle. Circulation. Sept 1994;90(3):1459-68.

39. Zipes DP, Rubart M. Neural modulation of cardiac arrhythmias and sudden cardiac death. Heart Rhythm. Jan 2006;3(1):108-13.

40. Klocke FJ, Kaiser GA, Ross J, Braunwald E. An Intrinsic Adrenergic Vasodilator Mechanism in the Coronary Vascular Bed of the Dog. Circulation Research. Apr 1965;16(4):376-82.

41. Heusch G. The paradox of a-adrenergic coronary vasoconstriction revisited. Journal of Molecular and Cellular Cardiology. July 2011;51(1):16-23.

42. Komaru T, Lamping KG, Eastham CL, Harrison DG, Marcus ML, Dellsperger KC. Effect of an arginine analogue on acetylcholine-induced coronary microvascular dilatation in dogs. American Journal of Physiology-Heart and Circulatory Physiology. 1 Dec 1991;261(6):H2001-7.

43. Reid JV, Ito BR, Huang AH, Buffington CW, Feigl EO. Parasympathetic control of transmural coronary blood flow in dogs. American Journal of Physiology-Heart and Circulatory Physiology. August 1, 1985;249(2):H337-43.

44. Pelc LR, Gross GJ, Warltier DC. Changes in regional myocardial perfusion by muscarinic receptor subtypes in dogs. Cardiovascular Research. 1 July 1986;20(7):482-9.

45. Pelc LR, Daemmgen JW, Gross GJ, Warltier DC. Muscarinic

Receptor Subtypes Mediating Myocardial Blood Flow Redistribution: Journal of Cardiovascular Pharmacology. Apr 1988;11(4):424-31.

46. Zhang C, Knudson JD, Setty S, Araiza A, Dincer ÜD, Kuo L, et al. Coronary arteriolar vasoconstriction to angiotensin II is augmented in prediabetic metabolic syndrome via activation of AT 1 receptors. American Journal of Physiology-Heart and Circulatory Physiology. May 2005;288(5):H2154-62.

47. Myers PR, Banitt PF, Guerra R, Harrison DG. Characteristics of canine coronary resistance arteries: importance of endothelium. American Journal of Physiology-Heart and Circulatory Physiology. August 1, 1989;257(2):H603-10.

48. Katusic ZS, Shepherd JT, Vanhoutte PM. Vasopressin causes endothelium-dependent relaxations of the canine basilar artery. Circ Res. Nov 1984;55(5):575-9.

49. Nakayama K. Differential Contractile Responses of Pressurized Porcine Coronary Resistance-Sized and Conductance Coronary Arteries to Acetylcholine, Histamine and Prostaglandin F2".

50. Ginsburg R, Bristow MR, Davis K. Receptor mechanisms in the human epicardial coronary artery. Heterogeneous pharmacological response to histamine and carbachol. Circ Res. Sept 1984;55(3):416-21.

51. Hilton R, Eichholtz F. The influence of chemical factors on the coronary circulation. The Journal of Physiology. March 31, 1925;59(6):413-25.

52. Jackson WF. Arteriolar oxygen reactivity: where is the sensor and what is the mechanism of action? The Journal of Physiology. 15 Sep 2016;594(18):5055-77.

53. Jackson WF. Arteriolar oxygen reactivity: where is the sensor? American Journal of Physiology-Heart and Circulatory Physiology. 1 Nov 1987;253(5):H1120-6.

54. Jackson WF, Duling BR. The oxygen sensitivity of hamster cheek pouch arterioles. In vitro and in situ studies. Circ Res. Oct 1983;53(4):515-25.

55. Konold P, Gebert G, Brecht K. The mechanical response of isolated

arteries to potassium. Experientia. March 1968;24(3):247-8.

56. Berne RM. Cardiac nucleotides in hypoxia: possible role in regulation of coronary blood flow. American Journal of Physiology-Legacy Content. 1 Feb 1963;204(2):317-22.

57. Bache RJ, Dai XZ, Schwartz JS, Homans DC. Role of adenosine in coronary vasodilation during exercise. Circ Res. Apr 1988;62(4):846-53.

58. Yada T, Richmond KN, Van Bibber R, Kroll K, Feigl EO. Role of adenosine in local metabolic coronary vasodilation. American Journal of Physiology-Heart and Circulatory Physiology. May 1, 1999;276(5):H1425-33.

59. Liu Y, Zhao H, Li H, Kalyanaraman B, Nicolosi AC, Gutterman DD. Mitochondrial Sources of H 2 O 2 Generation Play a Key Role in Flow-Mediated Dilation in Human Coronary Resistance Arteries. Circulation Research. 19 sept 2003;93(6):573-80.

60. Kuo L, Thengchaisri N, W. Hein T. Regulation of Coronary Vasomotor Function by Reactive Oxygen Species. Mol Med Ther [Internet]. 2012 [cited 27 March 2024];01(01). Available from: http://www.scitechnol.com/2324- 8769/2324-8769-1-101.php

61. Rogers PA, Dick GM, Knudson JD, Focardi M, Bratz IN, Swafford AN, et al. H 2 O 2 -induced redox-sensitive coronary vasodilation is mediated by 4-aminopyridine-sensitive K$^+$ channels. American Journal of Physiology-Heart and Circulatory Physiology. Nov 2006;291(5):H2473-82.

62. Furchgott RF, Zawadzki JV. The obligatory role of endothelial cells in the relaxation of arterial smooth muscle by acetylcholine. Nature. nov 1980;288(5789):373-6.

63. Ignarro LJ, Buga GM, Wood KS, Byrns RE, Chaudhuri G. Endothelium-derived relaxing factor produced and released from artery and vein is nitric oxide. Proc Natl Acad Sci USA. Dec 1987;84(24):9265-9.

64. Fôrstermann U, Closs EI, Pollock JS, Nakane M, Schwarz P, Gath I, et al. Nitric oxide synthase isozymes. Characterization, purification, molecular cloning, and functions. Hypertension. June

1994;23(6_pt_2):1121-31.

65. Moncada S, Palmer RM, Higgs EA. Nitric oxide: physiology, pathophysiology, and pharmacology. Pharmacol Rev. June 1991;43(2):109-42.

66. Dick GM, Tune JD. Role of potassium channels in coronary vasodilation. Exp Biol Med (Maywood). Jan 2010;235(1):10-22.

67. Durand MJ, Gutterman DD. Diversity in mechanisms of endothelium-dependent vasodilation in health and disease. Microcirculation. Apr 2013;20(3):239-47.

68. Beyer AM, Gutterman DD. Regulation of the human coronary microcirculation. Journal of Molecular and Cellular Cardiology. Apr 2012;52(4):814-21.

69. Dai XZ, Bache RJ. Effect of indomethacin on coronary blood flow during graded treadmill exercise in the dog. American Journal of Physiology-Heart and Circulatory Physiology. 1 Sep 1984;247(3):H452-8.

70. Gebremedhin D, Harder DR, Pratt PF, Campbell WB. Bioassay of an Endothelium-Derived Hyperpolarizing Factor from Bovine Coronary Arteries: Role of a Cytochrome P450 Metabolite. J Vasc Res. 1998;35(4):274-84.

71. Ellinsworth DC, Sandow SL, Shukla N, Liu Y, Jeremy JY, Gutterman DD. Endothelium-Derived Hyperpolarization and Coronary Vasodilation: Diverse and Integrated Roles of Epoxyeicosatrienoic Acids, Hydrogen Peroxide, and Gap Junctions. Microcirculation. Jan 2016;23(1):15-32.

72. Edwards G, Dora KA, Gardener MJ, Garland CJ, Weston AH. K+ is an endothelium-derived hyperpolarizing factor in rat arteries. Nature. nov 1998;396(6708):269-72.

73. Batenburg WW, Popp R, Fleming I, Vries RD, Garrelds IM, Saxena PR, et al. Bradykinin-induced relaxation of coronary microarteries: S - nitrosothiols as EDHF? British J Pharmacology. May 2004;142(1):125-35.

74. Batenburg WW, De Vries R, Saxena PR, Jan Danser AH. L-S-Nitrosothiols: endothelium-derived hyperpolarizing factors in porcine

coronary arteries? Journal of Hypertension. Oct 2004;22(10):1927-36.

75. Yanagisawa M, Kurihara H, Kimura S, Goto K, Masaki T. A novel vasoconstrictor peptide, endothelin, is produced by vascular endothelium and modulates smooth muscle Ca2+ channels: Journal of Hypertension. Dec 1988;6(4):S188-191.

76. Rubanyi GM, Polokoff MA. Endothelins: molecular biology, biochemistry, pharmacology, physiology, and pathophysiology. Pharmacol Rev. Sept 1994;46(3):325-415.

77. Golino P, Ashton JH, Buja LM, Rosolowsky M, Taylor AL, McNatt J, et al. Local platelet activation causes vasoconstriction of large epicardial canine coronary arteries in vivo. Thromboxane A2 and serotonin are possible mediators. Circulation. Jan 1989;79(1):154-66.

78. Konidala S, Gutterman DD. Coronary vasospasm and the regulation of coronary blood flow. Progress in Cardiovascular Diseases. Jan 2004;46(4):349-73.

79. Matta A, Bouisset F, Lhermusier T, Campelo-Parada F, Elbaz M, Carrié D, et al. Coronary Artery Spasm: New Insights. Journal of Interventional Cardiology. May 15, 2020;2020:1-10.

80. Montone RA, Niccoli G, Fracassi F, Russo M, Gurgoglione F, Cammà G, et al. Patients with acute myocardial infarction and non-obstructive coronary arteries: safety and prognostic relevance of invasive coronary provocative tests. European Heart Journal [Internet]. 8 Dec 2017 [cited 30 Mar 2024]; Available from: http://academic.oup.com/eurheartj/advance-article/doi/10.1093/eurheartj/ehx667/4710061

81. Bugiardini R, Manfrini O, De Ferrari GM. Unanswered Questions for Management of Acute Coronary Syndrome: Risk Stratification of Patients With Minimal Disease or Normal Findings on Coronary Angiography. Arch Intern Med. 10 Jul 2006;166(13):1391.

82. Planer D, Mehran R, Ohman EM, White HD, Newman JD, Xu K, et al. Prognosis of Patients With Non-ST-Segment-Elevation Myocardial Infarction and Nonobstructive Coronary Artery Disease: Propensity-Matched Analysis From the Acute Catheterization and Urgent Intervention Triage Strategy Trial. Circ: Cardiovascular Interventions.

June 2014;7(3):285-93.

83. Ong P, Athanasiadis A, Hill S, Vogelsberg H, Voehringer M, Sechtem U. Coronary Artery Spasm as a Frequent Cause of Acute Coronary Syndrome. 2008;52(7).

84. Yasue H, Sasayama S, Kikuchi K. The study on the role of coronary spasm in ischemic heart disease. In: Annual report of the research on cardiovascular diseases. Osaka: National Cardiovascular Center,. 2000;96-7.

85. Hung M, Hsu K, Hung M, Cheng C, Cherng W. Interactions among gender, age, hypertension and C-reactive protein in coronary vasospasm. Eur J Clin Investigation. Dec 2010;40(12):1094-103.

86. Ohba K, Sugiyama S, Sumida H, Nozaki T, Matsubara J, Matsuzawa Y, et al. Microvascular Coronary Artery Spasm Presents Distinctive Clinical Features With Endothelial Dysfunction as Nonobstructive Coronary Artery Disease. JAHA. 26 Sep 2012;1(5):e002485.

87. Yaker ZS, Lincoff AM, Cho L, Ellis SG, Ziada KM, Zieminski JJ, et al. Coronary spasm and vasomotor dysfunction as a cause of MINOCA. EuroIntervention. Jan 2024;20(2):e123-34.

88. Pristipino C, Beltrame JF, Finocchiaro ML, Hattori R, Fujita M, Mongiardo R, et al. Major Racial Differences in Coronary Constrictor Response Between Japanese and Caucasians With Recent Myocardial Infarction. Circulation. March 14, 2000;101(10):1102-8.

89. Nam P, Choi BG, Choi SY, Byun JK, Mashaly A, Park Y, et al. The impact of myocardial bridge on coronary artery spasm and long-term clinical outcomes in patients without significant atherosclerotic stenosis. Atherosclerosis. March 2018;270:8-12.

90. Sara JDS, Corban MT, Prasad M, Prasad A, Gulati R, Lerman LO, et al. Prevalence of myocardial bridging associated with coronary endothelial dysfunction in patients with chest pain and non-obstructive coronary artery disease. EuroIntervention. Feb 2020;15(14):1262-8.

91. Knuuti J. 2019 ESC Guidelines for the diagnosis and management of chronic coronary syndromes The Task Force for the diagnosis and management of chronic coronary syndromes of the European Society of

Cardiology (ESC). Russ J Cardiol. March 11, 2020;25(2):119-80.

92. Yasue H, Kugiyama K. Coronary Spasm: Clinical Features and Pathogenesis. Intern Med. 1997;36(11):760-5.

93. Rosamond W. Are Migraine and Coronary Heart Disease Associated? An Epidemiologic Review.Headache [Internet]. May 2004 [cited 22Apr 2024];44(s1).Available at: https://headachejournal.onlinelibrary.wiley.com/doi/10.1111/j.1526-4610.2004.04103.x

94. Stern S, Bayes De Luna A. Coronary Artery Spasm: A 2009 Update. Circulation. 12 May 2009;119(18):2531-4.

95. Sugiishi M, Takatsu F. Cigarette smoking is a major risk factor for coronary spasm. Circulation. Jan 1993;87(1):76-9.

96. Lin Z, Lin X, Zhao X, Xu C, Yu B, Shen Y, et al. Coronary Artery Spasm: Risk Factors, Pathophysiological Mechanisms and Novel Diagnostic Approaches. Rev Cardiovasc Med. 16 May 2022;23(5):175.

97. Ambrose JA, Barua RS. The pathophysiology of cigarette smoking and cardiovascular disease. Journal of the American College of Cardiology. May 2004;43(10):1731-7.

98. Ong P, Carro A, Athanasiadis A, Borgulya G, Schaufele T, Ratge D, et al. Acetylcholine-induced coronary spasm in patients with unobstructed coronary arteries is associated with elevated concentrations of soluble CD40 ligand and high-sensitivity C-reactive protein. Coronary Artery Disease. March 2015;26(2):126-32.

99. Hung MJ, Hsu KH, Hu WS, Chang NC, Hung MY. C-Reactive Protein for Predicting Prognosis and Its Gender-Specific Associations with Diabetes. Mellitus and Hypertension in the Development of Coronary Artery Spasm. Aoki I, editor. PLoS ONE. 28 Oct 2013;8(10):e77655.

100. Takaoka K, Yoshimura M, Ogawa H, Kugiyama K, Nakayama M, Shimasaki Y, et al. Comparison of the risk factors for coronary artery spasm with those for organic stenosis in a Japanese population: role of cigarette smoking. International Journal of Cardiology. Jan 2000;72(2):121-6.

101. Li YJ, Hyun MH, Rha SW, Chen KY, Jin Z, Dang Q, et al. Diabetes

mellitus is not a risk factor for coronary artery spasm as assessed by an intracoronary acetylcholine provocation test: angiographic and clinical characteristics of 986 patients. J Invasive Cardiol. June 2014;26(6):234-9.

102. Kawahara J, Kaku B, Yagi K, Kitagawa N, Yokoyama M, Wakabayashi Y, et al. Life-threatening coronary vasospasm in patients with type 2 diabetes with SGLT2 inhibitor-induced euglycemic ketoacidosis: a report of two consecutive cases. Diabetol Int. Jan 2024;15(1):135-40.

103. Hung MJ, Chang NC, Hu P, Chen TH, Mao CT, Yeh CT, et al. Association between Coronary Artery Spasm and the risk of incident Diabetes: A Nationwide population-based Cohort Study. Int J Med Sci. 2021;18(12):2630-40.

104. Raizner AE, Chahine RA, Ishimori T, Verani MS, Zacca N, Jamal N, et al. Provocation of coronary artery spasm by the cold pressor test. Hemodynamic, arteriographic and quantitative angiographic observations. Circulation. nov 1980;62(5):925-32.

105. Yasue H, Omote S, Takizawa A, Nagao M, Miwa K, Tanaka S. Circadian variation of exercise capacity in patients with Prinzmetal's variant angina: role of exercise-induced coronary arterial spasm. Circulation. May 1979;59(5):938-48.

106. Yeung AC, Vekshtein VI, Krantz DS, Vita JA, Ryan TJ, Ganz P, et al. The Effect of Atherosclerosis on the Vasomotor Response of Coronary Arteries to Mental Stress. N Engl J Med. 28 Nov 1991;325(22):1551-6.

107. Nakao K, Ohgushi M, Yoshimura M, Morooka K, Okumura K, Ogawa H, et al. Hyperventilation as a Specific Test for Diagnosis of Coronary Artery Spasm. The American Journal of Cardiology. Sept 1997;80(5):545-9.

108. Miyagi H, Yasue H, Okumura K, Ogawa H, Goto K, Oshima S. Effect of magnesium on anginal attack induced by hyperventilation in patients with variant angina. Circulation. March 1989;79(3):597-602.

109. Takizawa A, Yasue H, Omote S, Nagao M, Hyon H, Nishida S, et al. Variant angina induced by alcohol ingestion. American Heart Journal.

Jan 1984;107(1):25-7.

110. Robertson RM, Bernard Y, Robertson D. Arterial and coronary sinus catecholamines in the course of spontaneous coronary artery spasm. American Heart Journal. June 1983;105(6):901-6.

111. Yasue H, Horio Y, Nakamura N, Fujii H, Imoto N, Sonoda R, et al. Induction of coronary artery spasm by acetylcholine in patients with variant angina: possible role of the parasympathetic nervous system in the pathogenesis of coronary artery spasm. Circulation. nov 1986;74(5):955-63.

112. J. R. Lewis, R. Kisilevsky, P. W. Armstrong. Prinzmetal's angina, normal coronary arteries and pericarditis. CMAJ. July 8, 1978;119(1):36.

113. Forman MB, Oates JA, Robertson D, Robertson RM, Roberts LJ, Virmani R. Increased Adventitial Mast Cells in a Patient with Coronary Spasm. N Engl J Med. 31 Oct 1985;313(18):1138-41.

114. Shimokawa H. Cellular and Molecular Mechanisms of Coronary Artery Spasm: - Lessons From Animal Models -. Jpn Circ J. 2000;64(1):1-12.

115. Hung MJ, Cherng WJ, Cheng CW, Li LF. Comparison of Serum Levels of Inflammatory Markers in Patients With Coronary Vasospasm Without Significant Fixed Coronary Artery Disease Versus Patients With Stable Angina Pectoris and Acute Coronary Syndromes With Significant Fixed Coronary Artery Disease. The American Journal of Cardiology. May 2006;97(10):1429-34.

116. Itoh T, Mizuno Y, Harada E, Yoshimura M, Ogawa H, Yasue H. Coronary Spasm is Associated With Chronic Low-Grade Inflammation. Circ J. 2007;71(7):1074-8.

117. Hung MJ, Cherng WJ, Hung MY, Kuo LT, Cheng CW, Wang CH, et al. Increased leukocyte Rho-associated coiled-coil containing protein kinase activity predicts the presence and severity of coronary vasospastic angina. Atherosclerosis. Apr 2012;221(2):521-6.

118. Shimokawa H. 2014 Williams Harvey Lecture: importance of coronary vasomotion abnormalities--from bench to bedside. European Heart Journal. 1 Dec 2014;35(45):3180-93.

119. Feenstra RGT, Boerhout CKM, Woudstra J, Vink CEM, Wittekoek ME, De Waard GA, et al. Presence of Coronary Endothelial Dysfunction, Coronary Vasospasm, and Adenosine-Mediated Vasodilatory Disorders in Patients With Ischemia and Nonobstructive Coronary Arteries. Circ: Cardiovascular Interventions [Internet]. August 2022 [cited 25 Apr 2024];15(8). Available sur: https://www.ahajournals.org/doi/10.1161/CIRCINTERVENTIONS.122.012017

120. Yasue H, Mizuno Y, Harada E. Coronary artery spasm – Clinical features, pathogenesis and treatment –. Proceedings of the Japan Academy Ser B: Physical and Biological Sciences. Feb 8, 2019;95(2):53-66.

121. Lanza GA, Careri G, Crea F. Mechanisms of Coronary Artery Spasm. Circulation. 18 Oct 2011;124(16):1774-82.

122. Masumoto A, Mohri M, Shimokawa H, Urakami L, Usui M, Takeshita A. Suppression of Coronary Artery Spasm by the Rho-Kinase Inhibitor Fasudil in Patients With Vasospastic Angina. Circulation. 2 Apr 2002;105(13):1545-7.

123. Shimokawa H. Rho-kinase-mediated pathway induces enhanced myosin light chain phosphorylations in a swine model of coronary artery spasm. Cardiovascular Research. sept 1999;43(4):1029-39.

124. Hubert A, Seitz A, Pereyra VM, Bekeredjian R, Sechtem U, Ong P. Coronary Artery Spasm: The Interplay Between Endothelial Dysfunction and Vascular Smooth Muscle Cell Hyperreactivity. European Cardiology Review [Internet]. Feb 2020 [cited 25 Apr 2024];15. Available from: https://www.ncbi.nlm.nih.gov/pmc/articles/PMC7199189/

125. Kaski JC, Maseri A, Vejar M, Crea F, Hackett D. Spontaneous coronary artery spasm in variant angina is caused by a local hyperreactivity to a generalized constrictor stimulus. J Am Coll Cardiol. 15 Nov 1989;14(6):1456-63.

126. Sharma P, Jha AB, Dubey RS, Pessarakli M. Reactive Oxygen Species, Oxidative Damage, and Antioxidative Defense Mechanism in Plants under Stressful Conditions. Journal of Botany. 24 Apr 2012;2012:e217037.

127. Franczyk B, Dybiec J, Frqk W, Krzemir'ska J, Kuémierz J, Mfynarska E, et al. Cellular Mechanisms of Coronary Artery Spasm. Biomedicines. 21 Sep 2022;10(10):2349.

128. Pahimi N, Rasool AHG, Sanip Z, Bokti NA, Yusof Z, W. Isa WYH. An Evaluation of the Role of Oxidative Stress in Non-Obstructive Coronary Artery Disease. J Cardiovasc Dev Dis. 4 Feb 2022;9(2):51.

129. Chistiakov DA, Melnichenko AA, Grechko AV, Myasoedova VA, Orekhov AN. Potential of anti-inflammatory agents for treatment of atherosclerosis. Experimental and Molecular Pathology. Apr 2018;104(2):114-24.

130. Xu S, Ilyas I, Little PJ, Li H, Kamato D, Zheng X, et al. Endothelial Dysfunction in Atherosclerotic Cardiovascular Diseases and Beyond: From Mechanism to Pharmacotherapies. Ma Q, editor. Pharmacol Rev. Jul 2021;73(3):924-67.

131. Yamagishi M, Miyatake K, Tamai J, Nakatani S, Koyama J, Nissen SE. Intravascular ultrasound detection of atherosclerosis at the site of focal vasospasm in angiographically normal or minimally narrowed coronary segments. Journal of the American College of Cardiology. Feb 1994;23(2):352-7.

132. Pellegrini D, Konst R, Van Den Oord S, Dimitriu-Leen A, Mol JQ, Jansen T, et al. Features of atherosclerosis in patients with angina and no obstructive coronary artery disease. EuroIntervention. August 2022;18(5):e397-404.

133. Shin DI, Baek SH, Her SH, Han SH, Ahn Y, Park KH, et al. The 24-Month Prognosis of Patients With Positive or Intermediate Results in the Intracoronary Ergonovine Provocation Test. JACC: Cardiovascular Interventions. June 2015;8(7):914-23.

134. Slavich M, Patel RS. Coronary artery spasm: Current knowledge and residual uncertainties. IJC Heart & Vasculature. March 2016;10:47-53.

135. Oshima S, Yasue H, Ogawa H, Okumura K, Matsuyama K. Fibrinopeptide A is released into the coronary circulation after coronary spasm. Circulation. Dec 1990;82(6):2222-5.

136. Ogawa H, Yasue H, Oshima S, Okumura K, Matsuyama K, Obata K. Circadian variation of plasma fibrinopeptide A level in patients with variant angina. Circulation. Dec 1989;80(6):1617-26.

137. Miyamoto S, Ogawa H, Soejima H, Takazoe K, Sakamoto T, Yoshimura M, et al. Formation of platelet aggregates after attacks of coronary spastic angina pectoris. The American Journal of Cardiology. Feb 2000;85(4):494-7.

138. Goto K, Yasue H, Okumura K, Matsuyama K, Kugiyama K, Miyagi H, et al. Magnesium deficiency detected by intravenous loading test in variant angina pectoris. The American Journal of Cardiology. March 1990;65(11):709-12.

139. Hung MJ, Hu P, Hung MY. Coronary Artery Spasm: Review and Update. Int J Med Sci. 2014;11(11):1161-71.

140. Kounis NG, Zavras GM. HISTAMINE-INDUCED CORONARY ARTERY SPASM: THE CONCEPT OF ALLERGIC ANGINA. Int J Clinical Practice. June 1991;45(2):121-8.

141. Sakata K, Iida K, Kudo M, Yoshida H, Doi O. Prognostic Value of I-123 Metaiodobenzylguanidine Imaging in Vasospastic Angina Without Significant Coronary Stenosis. Circ J. 2005;69(2):171-6.

142. Camici PG, d'Amati G, Rimoldi O. Coronary microvascular dysfunction: mechanisms and functional assessment. Nat Rev Cardiol. Jan 2015;12(1):48-62.

143. Ong P, Athanasiadis A, Mahrholdt H, Shah BN, Sechtem U, Senior R. Transient Myocardial Ischemia During Acetylcholine-Induced Coronary Microvascular Dysfunction Documented by Myocardial Contrast Echocardiography. Circ: Cardiovascular Imaging. Jan 2013;6(1):153-5.

144. Ong P, Athanasiadis A, Borgulya G, Vokshi I, Bastiaenen R, Kubik S, et al. Clinical Usefulness, Angiographic Characteristics, and Safety Evaluation of Intracoronary Acetylcholine Provocation Testing Among 921 Consecutive White Patients With Unobstructed Coronary Arteries. Circulation. Apr 29, 2014;129(17):1723-30.

145. Beltrame JF, Crea F, Kaski JC, Ogawa H, Ong P, Sechtem U, et al.

International standardization of diagnostic criteria for vasospastic angina. Eur Heart J. August 4, 2015;ehv351.

146. Tanaka A, Shimada K, Tearney GJ, Kitabata H, Taguchi H, Fukuda S, et al. Conformational Change in Coronary Artery Structure Assessed by Optical Coherence Tomography in Patients With Vasospastic Angina. Journal of the American College of Cardiology. Oct 2011;58(15):1608-13.

147. Shin ES, Ann SH, Singh GB, Lim KH, Yoon HJ, Hur SH, et al. OCT-Defined Morphological Characteristics of Coronary Artery Spasm Sites in Vasospastic Angina. JACC: Cardiovascular Imaging. sept 2015;8(9):1059-67.

148. Choi BG, Rha SW, Park T, Choi SY, Byun JK, Shim MS, et al. Impact of Cigarette Smoking: a 3-Year Clinical Outcome of Vasospastic Angina Patients. Korean Circ J. 2016;46(5):632.

149. Mizuno Y, Harada E, Morita S, Kinoshita K, Hayashida M, Shono M, et al. East Asian Variant of Aldehyde Dehydrogenase 2 Is Associated With Coronary Spastic Angina: Possible Roles of Reactive Aldehydes and Implications of Alcohol Flushing Syndrome. Circulation. May 12, 2015;131(19):1665-73.

150. Chu G, Zhang G, Zhang Z, Liu S, Wen Q, Sun B. Clinical Outcome of Coronary Stenting in Patients with Variant Angina Refractory to Medical Treatment: A Consecutive Single-Center Analysis. Med Princ Pract. 2013;22(6):583-7.

151. Lin Y, Liu H, Yu D, Wu M, Liu Q, Liang X, et al. Sympathectomy versus conventional treatment for refractory coronary artery spasm. Coronary Artery Disease. Sep 2019;30(6):418-24.

152. Elbadawi A, Elgendy IY, Naqvi SY, Mohamed AH, Ogunbayo GO, Omer MA, et al. Temporal Trends and Outcomes of Hospitalizations With Prinzmetal Angina: Perspectives From a National Database. The American Journal of Medicine. Sep 2019;132(9):1053-1061.e1.

153. Takagi Y, Yasuda S, Tsunoda R, Ogata Y, Seki A, Sumiyoshi T, et al. Clinical Characteristics and Long-Term Prognosis of Vasospastic Angina Patients Who Survived Out-of-Hospital Cardiac Arrest: Multicenter Registry Study of the Japanese Coronary Spasm

Association. Circ: Arrhythmia and Electrophysiology. June 2011;4(3):295-302.

154. Waters DD, Miller DD, Szlachcic J, Bouchard A, Méthé M, Kreeft J, et al. Factors influencing the long-term prognosis of treated patients with variant angina. Circulation. August 1983;68(2):258-65.

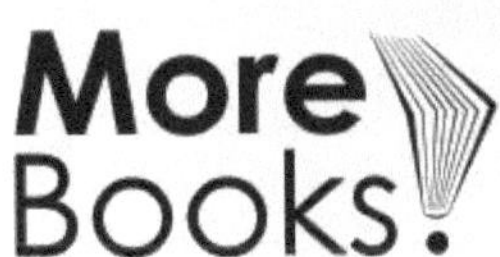

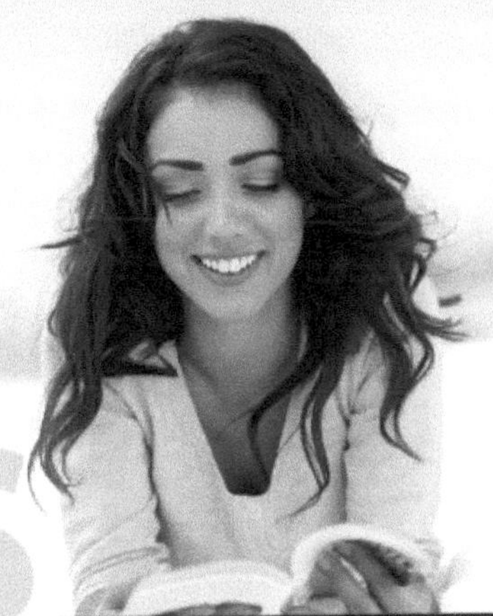

yes

I want morebooks!

Buy your books fast and straightforward online - at one of world's fastest growing online book stores! Environmentally sound due to Print-on-Demand technologies.

Buy your books online at
www.morebooks.shop

Kaufen Sie Ihre Bücher schnell und unkompliziert online – auf einer der am schnellsten wachsenden Buchhandelsplattformen weltweit! Dank Print-On-Demand umwelt- und ressourcenschonend produziert.

Bücher schneller online kaufen
www.morebooks.shop

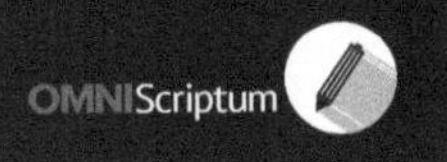

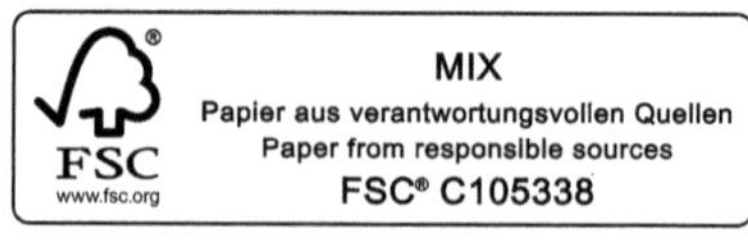

Printed by Books on Demand GmbH, Norderstedt / Germany